"Trust Me, I'm a Doctor"

NO! DON'T TRUST
ME! IT'S JUST
A JOKE!

Mark Depaolis

"Trust Me, I'm a Doctor"

*Humorous Second Opinions
for Everyday Life*

MARK DEPAOLIS

FAIRVIEW PRESS   *Minneapolis*

The contents of this book previously have appeared in the *Star Tribune* of Minneapolis-St. Paul and are reprinted with permission.

Published by Fairview Press, 2450 Riverside Avenue South, Minneapolis, MN 55454.

Library of Congress Cataloging-in-Publication Data

DePaolis, Mark, 1956-
    "Trust me, I'm a doctor" : humorous second opinions for everyday life / Mark DePaolis.
        p.   cm.
    ISBN 0-925190-39-X : 10.95
    1. Medicine—Humor.   I. Title.
    PN6231.M4D47   1995
    818'.5402—dc20   95-3180
                                                                                            CIP

First Printing: March 1995

Printed in the United States of America
99 98 97 96 95   7 6 5 4 3 2 1

Cover design: Circus Design
Cover photo: Mowers Photography

Publisher's Note: Fairview Press publishes books and other materials related to the subjects of physical health, mental health, and chemical dependency. Its publications, including *Trust Me, I'm a Doctor,* do not necessarily reflect the philosophy of Fairview Hospital and Healthcare Services or their treatment programs.

The paper used in this publication meets the minimum requirements of American National Standards for Information Sciences—Permanence of Paper for Printed Library Materials, ANSI Z329.48-1984.

To my parents, who made me

believe I could do anything,

and to my wife,

who married me and

proved their point

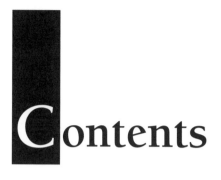

Contents

Acknowledgments

Thanks to Maureen LaJoy, who used her Three Rules to get me writing again, and to Vicki Palmquist, who kept me going with emotional and technical support.

And also to Glen Griffin at *Postgraduate Medicine,* who gave me my big break, and to editor Sandra Hoyt, who treated me like a writer, not a doctor.

A special thanks to my editor at the *Star Tribune,* Eric Ringham, who has the same twisted sense of humor and decided to take a chance on me. Thanks also to Robert White, who let him do it, and to Susan Albright, who continues to let him do it.

And I want to thank my wife, Rosa Marroquin, who has the most important job of all: reminding me that not everything is funny.

Introduction
"What Kind of a Doctor Are You?"

A book like this doesn't just write itself. I had to write it, although not all at the same time. Most of it was written piece by piece over the last three years. Each piece was a newspaper column called "Second Opinion," which appears in the Minneapolis *Star Tribune,* the newspaper of the Twin Cities.

There I write about medical topics as they relate to normal humans, instead of doctors. Although "Second Opinion" is a humor column, it has always been my greatest secret joy to sneak in some actual medical information between references to cartoon characters and space aliens. Because of this my column appears on the editorial page, right next to important articles about politics and world peace.

A lot of people wonder how it works being both a doctor and a writer. They can't believe I can have two different careers. They wonder how I have time to keep up on the latest advances in medicine as well as current trends in Mighty Morphin Power Rangers and fat-free snack foods.

Actually, I think it works best to combine the two.

While in the office I carry a stethoscope and wear a white coat, just like any doctor. The difference is that after taking care of some-one's pneumonia or skin problem I will duck into the next room and quickly knock out a few paragraphs of my latest column. I might perform a minor surgical operation, like removing a cyst, and then (after a thorough washing) do a quick rewrite on a particularly moving passage containing a joke about mucous.

While complicated, this system generally works for me. In fact, the two jobs are not all that different. There are considerable areas of overlap, as shown in this handy chart:

DOCTORING	WRITING
adnexal mass	adjective clause
foreskin	foreword
letters from	columns about
obnoxious lawyers	obnoxious lawyers
appendix	appendix

As you can see, the work is really very similar. In fact, sometimes it is hard to keep the two separate. Normally I can keep it straight, although I occasionally find myself diagnosing an editor or scribbling a few notes on someone's internal organs.

This arrangement also makes it easy to answer the question that everyone always asks writers, which is "Where do you get your ideas?" Many of them come from my patients.

I encourage my patients to ask questions. If I have learned anything in medicine, it's that if one person wants an answer, probably a lot of others are wondering the same thing. That's why I always try to give people the best, most plausible answer I can think of at the time, which is often "it's a virus." Then I quickly run to the next room and make up some jokes about doctors who think viruses cause everything.

This way if I am able to put just one person's mind at ease, while getting a column out of it besides, I feel I am doing my jobs.

If my patients only knew—which of course they will, because I will be prescribing a copy of this book for a variety of medical problems from now on.

I sometimes worry what patients might think when they see their doctor's name in the paper, especially when the name is accompanied by a photo that looks more like Sebastian Cabot. So far, the response has been just fine. I even get new patients this way. They come to me for various reasons: because they like what I write; because they appreciate my humorous, common-sense approach to medicine; or because they think I can get them a discount subscription. Still, over the last three years I have heard one overwhelming response from patients, which is: "What column?" This proves that you are never as famous as you think you are.

Other doctors have been supportive of the column, too, although some of them believe that I must have gone to medical school in some other, far-off place, such as the planet Wongo. While they may not agree with everything I say, many of them tell me they are glad someone is saying it. Oh, there are a few doctors who would prefer that I keep these medical things secret, but if that's the way they feel then they should never have given me my doctor's club secret decoder ring.

Besides, it's not just me. A lot of doctors are funny. Maybe not laughing-out-loud, squirt-milk-out-your-nose funny, but certainly quite amusing. I know many doctors who can really crack you up, especially at 3:30 a.m. while you're eating strained peaches from the pediatric ward when you are so tired you go into hysterics every time someone says the word "coccyx."

Unfortunately, most people don't know this. They imagine I am different, that I must work in some bizarre, humor-related medical specialty, like Laughter Therapy or Gigglolgy. This is reassuring to them; they think that this way they are less likely to find me looking at them from across a hospital bed.

Naturally, there is a lot about medicine that is serious business. But there are also a lot of things that are funny. Laughing helps me to be a better doctor.

It's kind of like wearing a goofy tie. A colorful, exotic tie used to be a sign that someone was a cretin, but silly ties have become, as of this writing, the standard uniform of every middle-age business man. At meetings in Fortune 500 corporations you can see older men in dark gray suits wearing ties the color of highway warning signs, often featuring pictures of Tweety Bird or R2D2.

Being a funny doctor is like that. Of course, on any given day not

3

everyone will be in the mood for cartoons, but most people notice and appreciate them. If not, they generally only see a tie.

By now, the question on your mind is obvious: If a lot of doctors are funny and there is nothing special about me, why do I get to write a newspaper column and, subsequently, a book?

I have been considering this question for the last few years. Considering current directions in health care, taking into account the decline of the solo practitioner and the trend toward large mergers, and factoring in the genuine desire of most doctors to help patients and all humankind, I believe there is really only one answer:

Because I thought of it first.

Practice Makes Perfect

I love practicing medicine. My plan is to keep practicing until I get it right; then I'll retire.

All doctors are just practicing. They'll tell you so if you ask them. It makes you wonder how there can be so many malpractice suits—after all, we're only practicing. It's not like we claimed to be perfect or anything.

The key to successful practice is to know the rules. Unfortunately, doctors have been forbidden to share these rules with the general public . . . until now.

The Cold Facts about Viruses

Let's take a look at one of the most important questions facing health care consumers, which is, "What the heck is the doctor looking at with that little flashlight, anyway?"

No matter what season, people are always coming down with "communal respiratory ubiquitous disease (CRUD)." Many people will be going to the doctor's office with this virus soon, more than once if they have children, and it is good to know what to expect when you get there.

The visit begins with the nurse, who will take your temperature and ask a variety of questions about how long you have been sick, what the symptoms are, and any medications you might be taking. She (or he) writes the answers on the chart, and then asks you to undress and step into a lush, full-length dressing gown of soft cotton with satin trim.

Next the doctor comes in, carrying the same chart. He (or she) asks you some questions about how long you have been sick, what the symptoms are, and any medications you might be taking. If it is your regular doctor, he might also ask about your vacation to Disney World last summer.

The exam then begins. The doctor asks you to sit on a tall, comfortable, divan-type sofa that has been reupholstered in butcher paper. He then takes a flashlight and begins to look into various openings in your head.

The eyes come first, because they always come first. Some doctors pull down the lids to look at the soft, fleshy part underneath. This area can provide important clues to many problems, like whether any dirt got in there.

Next are the ears. Doctors already know that your ears hurt, because this happens no matter what is wrong with you. A broken

6

ankle can make your ears feel "kind of plugged." Many people cough when someone looks in their ears. This is a well-recognized phenomenon, caused by the proximity of the auditory canal to a branch of the cranial nerve called . . . well, I forget, but they're really close together in there, and somehow that makes you cough. Then he will feel your neck for lumps. This is very important, as any mother knows, because lumps can tell you if someone is really sick or just faking to get out of school. Now he tells you to open your mouth, shining the light in there and looking around. Most respiratory problems are caused by viruses, but they are too tiny to see, even with a really bright light. Fortunately for medical science, they also tend to be very messy. Viruses never wipe their feet or clean up after themselves, so you can usually see the mess they leave behind. This generally takes the form of gross, sickening white gobs. The doctor checks for gobs on the cheeks, the tonsils, and that thing hanging down in the back, called the "uvula" (from the latin Uvulatum, or "hangy thing doctors care about"). He also checks the tongue, which is supposed to have those big bumps in the back, and yes, they have always been there, and they are normal.

Next he listens to your back, which makes no sense because everyone knows all the really important organs are in the front. Remember how everything came tumbling out when you pulled the clear plastic stomach off the Visible Man doll you had in grade school? Actually, a trained physician can hear parts of the lungs back there, plus it gives him a chance to think without someone looking at him all the time.

Finally, he listens to your heart, which is pumping away like always. Hearts are like CEOs of major corporations, just too darn busy to worry about some little cold.

Fortunately, most of the time the examination is normal. The ears are OK, the throat has a few gobs but not too many, and the lungs are clear. The heart is too busy to be examined, but has promised to get back to you. With these reassuring findings, the doctor can then determine the precise cause of the illness. "It's a virus-type infection thing," he tells you. "Should run its course. Unless of course it gets worse, and then we can run 'some tests.' "

This veiled threat convinces the viruses to leave your body. Soon they will be catching the 5:15 sneeze to the person next to you on the bus, and you will start to feel better.

The visit is over. You can now get dressed and head home again, handing your gown to the valet on the way out. You are glad to know that you will soon be back to normal. As a special bonus, thanks to your doctor and your own natural antibodies, you will never be bothered with this particular virus again.

Lucky you—that only leaves 758,433,792 other strains to worry about.

Life's Little Emergencies

Quick—what's the official medical treatment for a folded ear?

Chances are you don't know, and that's because your doctor never had a chance to tell you about some pesky, everyday medical problems.

Medicine can tell you everything you want to know about Western Equine Panencephalitis, but it can be a little hazy when it comes to the pain you get on the roof of your mouth from eating ice cream.

Besides, visiting the doctor is just too much trouble. No one wants to make an appointment, spend half an hour in the waiting room, put on a white gown and then tell the nurse, "I just wanted to ask about those big bumps on the back of my tongue."

Instead, most people bring up these questions when they go to the doctor for some other reason, like a broken leg. While the doctor is busy setting the bone, the patient is trying to casually work in a question about those tiny pouches of skin in the armpits.

While I'm not saying that people are intentionally breaking bones just for a chance to ask questions, I am presenting a simple guide to some of these common, annoying medical problems, just so I can sleep at night:

Funny bone trauma

The ulnar nerve runs through a groove in the elbow, and banging it sends a shock wave through the nerve to the fingers, making them tingle. Nothing about this is funny. While most doctors understand this condition, it is hard for them to explain because several Latin terms are necessary to describe it. Official treatment is to stop banging it on things.

Eye-twitching

Twitching near the corner of the eye is harder to understand, although it is fair to say that very few of these cases are caused by secret radio transmissions from alien spacecraft urging us to break into NORAD command centers and deactivate the nuclear defense grid. Sometimes it's just nerves.

Folded ear

You awaken from sleep and suddenly realize that you are lying on your ear, which is plastered forward against the side of your head. The slightest move and it will snap back into place, causing blinding, searing pain that makes childbirth seem like minor indigestion.

Some people have been known to lie still for days, but the only real treatment is to lift your head, massage the ear vigorously once you regain consciousness and then splint it back in place for a few days with masking tape. Earmuffs can prevent relapses.

Limbs falling asleep

This condition is often misunderstood. Arms and legs do not actually fall asleep, but suffer a form of death, although generally a mild case.

No one knows how the limbs are brought back to life merely by shaking them and whispering, "Wake up, wake up," although this certainly has implications for the entire field of mortuary science.

Glass-sucking

Doctors don't really know what to do when someone is sucking on a drinking glass and it gets stuck to their face. Often they resort to "running a few tests" while their nurse calls a plumber.

They also have no idea what to do about the large, red splotch that encircles the patient's mouth for the remainder of the seventh grade, making it look as though their date for the big spring dance was a bathroom plunger.

Stubbed toe

Some people rush to the doctor after accidentally banging their little toe into the dresser, just because their toe quickly swells to the size of a mushy, purple golf ball and feels like a tea bag full of broken glass.

The doctor usually prescribes a block of wood to strap onto the foot, on the medical theory that people in pain should also look ridiculous. The only other recommended treatment is to scream a loud obscenity while using the other foot to kick the dresser, which can often be done at home.

Paper cuts

You treat these minor lacerations as you would any other cuts, gently scrubbing them with antibacterial soap and applying a clean, dry bandage. Paper cuts on the tongue, such as you get from licking envelopes, naturally require a different treatment; these do not need scrubbing before applying the bandage.

Floating spots

Many people have small dark spots that drift in and out of their fields of vision, looking like tiny, microscopic organisms performing water ballet. The official medical term for these, which is listed in many legitimate textbooks, is "floaters." They are normal.

There is one rare condition in which tiny parasitic worms can actually invade the eyeball and swim around, but luckily, most people don't know about it so they don't worry.

Explosive esophageal eruption

This occurs when you suffer a burp and a hiccup at the same

time, causing you to emit a loud noise and making you feel like someone used a boat hook to turn you inside out, giving nervous bystanders a look at vital internal organs.

There is no way to prevent these episodes. There is no treatment. There are no answers. Medicine has nothing to offer. Trust me— stick with the broken leg instead.

Stressed for Success

People today are under a lot of stress. Just turn on the news and you will see pictures of wars, hurricanes, budget deficits, and anchorpersons who have to keep their hair just perfect.

Stress affects everyone. I know a lot of you are just scanning these first few paragraphs because you saw the word "stress" in the title, wanting to read further but knowing you are just too darn busy.

That's OK. I understand. No sense wasting time reading about something you already know, mainly that you are under the kind of stress that is making your life frantic and is rapidly building to the point where you will soon burst into flames.

How do I know that people reading this are under stress? Because we all are. This is the '90s; stress has replaced "cynical idealism" as the dominant feeling of our time. The top-selling medicine in the country is for stomach ulcers. Our jobs are stressful, family life is stressful, reading articles about stress is stressful. Even if you don't think you are stressed out, you are. In fact, this may actually be the worst kind of stress, where you have the added stress of keeping it from yourself.

Stress wasn't always a bad thing. In earlier times, stress was due to the very real possibility of being eaten by wolves. Our ancestors learned to respond with surges of adrenaline, which allowed them to face the oncoming wolves and, in a sudden burst of incredible strength, push other people into their path. Nowadays, with wolf populations way down, this adrenaline only triggers a lot of senseless worrying. In a recent survey, about half of all people polled said that they worry so much that they are seriously worried about it, which is worrisome in itself.

This constant, nervous worrying leads to problems. There are many ways that stress can cause changes in your body. Eons from now I'm sure that humans will evolve special adaptations to stress, like thick armor plating inside their stomachs, but so far, most of these responses to stress are bad. Sooner or later, people under constant stress will become sick, and that's where doctors come in.

People often ask their doctors the question, "Could this be . . . stress?" Whatever the problem, the correct answer is always, "Of course." Headaches, back pain, fatigue, stomach upset, dizziness, depression—almost any physical complaint can be triggered by stress. Just asking the question means that the answer is probably "yes," even if the person just came in for a sprained ankle.

The real question is what to do about it. Most of the time we really can't eliminate all sources of stress unless we are willing to quit our jobs and move to deserted islands, and even then we would have to deal with mosquitoes and pesky tropical storms.

For another option watch one of those PBS specials with names like "Nature's Call of Wild Animal Adventure in Africa." Animals, you will notice, do not get stressed out. They sleep, they eat, they exercise, and that's pretty much it. They seem very calm, even those little antelopes that can be suddenly torn to bloody shreds at any moment by cheetahs, usually in full horrified view of my son. Living with this constant threat is several times more stressful than paying IRS late filing fees or taking kids to soccer practice, yet somehow they seem content.

Animals never start to twitch nervously or vomit unless some human puts them in a zoo, or worse, takes them home to live with them. Watch one of those little yapper dogs with manicured nails and bows on its ears, and try to imagine how quickly it would start complaining about tension headaches and tingling in its paws.

There is a message here for all of us. Eating better, getting enough sleep and exercising might be better than any medicine. Bill Clinton, the jogging president, only does one of the three, and he seems to be thriving. If you're well rested and in shape, the stresses of modern life won't matter quite as much.

At least you'll have the same chance as a small antelope. And, while you may have to face an occasional anchorperson, you are a lot less likely to run into a cheetah.

14

Do You Need a Physical?

People are always wondering whether they need physicals.

Unless you are over 60, doctors no longer recommend a physical exam every year, so the trick is to know when it is time. Otherwise, you run the risk of having a number of unpleasant things done to you for no good reason.

Do you really need to have a physical? Yes. Or, to put it another way, no. Actually, as with most things in medicine, it depends.

Let's say you are 50 years old and a chain smoker big enough to take up two seats on the bus. Your breathing isn't so good. You get splitting headaches every day when you leave the house. You can't eat solid food any more, and you get chest pains just from tying your shoes. Do you need a physical?

Obviously, the answer is no. For one thing, you would never make it to the appointment. Most physicals are scheduled months ahead, valuable time that you will need for cashing in bonds and selecting a funeral outfit. Any of these problems on its own is worth a visit to the doctor though, without waiting for an opening for a physical. Call now. Don't even let them put you on hold.

Here's another example: You are approaching 40 and have noticed a couple of disturbing changes going on in your body. You are no longer as fast as you once were. Your midsection is thicker than you remember, and your shoulders hurt a lot for no particular reason. Getting out of bed takes about 20 minutes, with care taken not to aggravate that pesky lower-back problem. Your vision is a little blurry when you read anything smaller than a license plate, and every so often you see the faint image of your long-dead grandfather standing silently next to your left elbow.

Time for a physical, you say? What for? Everybody feels like this. You are just getting older, and that's what any doctor will say.

They can tell because they're getting older, too.

Then how can you know when it is time to make an appointment? It depends on whether you are a man or a woman. Extensive medical research has shown that there is only one reliable sign that it is time for men to see a doctor, which is true in about 95 percent of cases: their wives make them go.

Women seem to have a better appreciation for medical science, particularly married women, who have a vested interest in how long their husbands are going to be around. Many of these men are sent to the doctor with a small slip of paper that says "I need a physical. Please tell me to lose weight and to stop watching so much ESPN. Thank you. Signed, My Wife."

Of course, not all men see doctors because of their wives. Sometimes their girlfriends or fiancées send them, with strict instructions to "get checked out" while there is still time to change the wedding plans. These women are smart—they know it is almost impossible to return a defective husband.

This is one reason that men get married. Someone has to help them take care of themselves. Men are not good at routine maintenance, except for outboard motors. Several research studies have been designed to investigate this difference between the sexes. Unfortunately, they have never been completed because the control groups of single men never survive long enough to show a trend.

Actually, this wife-directed system works pretty well. The best time to have a physical is when you feel fine, or, for most men, when they say they feel fine. That way the doctor can focus on the important points of their history, such as whether they consider "nachos" one of the four major food groups, or whether they count buying tires as a form of aerobic exercise.

What about women? How do they know when it is time to go to the doctor? I have no idea. Most of them need to come every year for pap smears (the highly secretive "female exam" they mentioned in eighth-grade hygiene class), and I'll be darned if they don't show up every year, sometimes to the exact day.

This knack for getting physicals at the proper time is one of the main reasons why women live longer than men, right up there along with their contempt for motorcycles and organized hockey.

Which is fine with most men. Being alive longer only means more physicals, more often, with even more unpleasant procedures. Many of them will tell you that if it weren't for their wives, it just wouldn't be worth it.

Shrinking Role of Psychiatrist's Couches

I have always been interested in psychotherapy, probably because I may one day need some. This field is full of startling discoveries, particularly in the area of therapeutic office furniture:

Startling Psychiatric Fact No. 1: It makes a big difference what kind of couch the therapist has

Couches have been a part of psychiatrists' offices ever since Freud. He believed his patients would feel freer to talk when lying down, even though medical research clearly shows that most people who are lying down are either asleep or dead. The real reason may have been to prevent them from seeing his facial expressions while they described their little problems with, for example, alpaca sweaters.

Sigmund's own couch of choice was a slender divan-type sofa, with an oriental rug thrown over it to keep hair off the upholstery.

Modern analysts also know the importance of office furniture, and they are careful to select the proper couch. According to a recent article in the *New York Times,* most of them opt for a neutral, unobtrusive color like beige or light gray, which doesn't show tear stains. Some choose large leather sofas, believing that leather has an aura of security and stability, although what it really provides is a sense of ex-cowness.

Others let their couches speak for them, especially since they never say much themselves besides "Um-hum." These therapists prefer couches in shocking colors or odd shapes. This can be confusing, and even painful, to patients who have trouble telling the furniture from other objects of art scattered around the office.

The point is that psychoanalysts believe their office couch is much more than just a piece of furniture, which is presumably how they also feel about cigars and certain elongated fruits. One thing they all agree on—a couch should not look too much like a bed. Sleeper sofas are definitely out.

Not content to merely report these research findings, I launched into some extensive research of my own, consisting primarily of a phone call to a friend who is a psychiatrist. He told me that the couch study is probably accurate, but that nobody is going to care because of—

Startling Psychiatric Fact No. 2: It doesn't matter, because very few psychiatrists have couches anymore anyway

Really! This is true. I know what you're thinking: How could thousands of made-for-TV movies be wrong? Psychiatrists turn up on TV all the time, and they always have couches in their offices. Could this all be part of some gigantic hoax?

Well, it turns out that psychiatrists used couches a lot more in the old days, but that strict Freudian analysis has pretty much gone the way of horse-drawn carriages and boom boxes without CD players.

My friend knew of only two psychiatrists who still have couches in their offices, and their patients use them for, if you can believe this, sitting down. The patients never lie down and stare at the ceiling like on TV, although sometimes they will try to re-create favorite scenes from "Days of Our Lives."

Clearly, the couch story is just another example of the way medical research can affect our daily lives, just a bit too late. In fact, the whole topic of analyst couches might be rendered moot thanks to—

Startling Psychiatric Fact No. 3: Some analysts don't have couches because they don't even have offices to put them in

According to a recent newspaper article, a local psychotherapist has started doing therapy over the phone, without any office at all.

Telephone Psychotherapy was started for those who are "just too busy or too sick" to make it to the office, but who can still find the time to be disturbed. It is also supposed to be helpful for people who have a fear of public places, although I expect it would take away their last real reason to leave the house.

The service has promised to send patients a photo of their therapist, looking concerned in a detached, nonjudgmental way, which they can then prop up behind them during the session. And of course, patients are free to lie down if they want to, although it might require a cordless.

Now, thanks to modern couch research, I will be able to keep these startling psychiatric breakthroughs in mind the next time I go shopping for a new couch myself. After all, I might need one some day. I hear light gray is nice.

Allergies in Season

Every year millions of people dread the onset of spring. For them, April means one thing: Ladies and gentlemen, start your allergies.

I'm glad I don't have allergies. Oh, sure, I do get a little stuffy around that time of year. I sneeze a bit more, my eyes tend to water, and my nose gets red enough to guide Santa's sleigh, but it's not from allergies. As a doctor, I can think of plenty of other reasons. I probably just have a cold, that's all, one that comes back for two months every year at precisely the same time.

The reason I know I don't have allergies is because I don't believe in them. I just can't accept that the human body, which routinely manufactures things like parathyroid hormone from scratch, can be unable to control its own nasal passages when spring comes.

People are the dominant organisms on the planet, as hardy as cockroaches and almost as smart as dolphins, and it's hard for me to believe we could be reduced to giant wheezing, sniffling mucous glands by mere household dust. This would require a major design flaw in the human blueprint, going against the basic medical principle that says most things get better, not worse, on their own.

So when I feel as if someone put sandpaper under my eyelids, and my head starts expanding like a pan of Jiffy Pop, I know it's probably just my sinuses. It will get better with a little saline spray (I use straight contact lens solution—none of that wimpy mist for me) and one of those heating pads shaped like a Darth Vader mask.

I'm glad, because if I had allergies I would have to take allergy medicine. Between over-the-counter and prescription products, there are roughly 366,783 different brands of allergy medicine, which can be divided into two groups:

Allergy medicines you can buy at convenience stores. These pills work very well to relieve symptoms, including the symptoms of

21

awareness and conscious thought. While asleep you feel great, but the symptoms return when you wake up with your head on your desk in a puddle of drool.

Allergy medicines you have to get from a doctor. These also work well to relieve symptoms, some without causing drooling or a coma, and all at no more cost than a vacation in Barbados, where they have never even seen household dust.

Of course, these medicines require you to call your doctor for a prescription. Some doctors, particularly if they believe in allergies, will do this over the phone. Others want you to come to the office so they can perform an accurate allergy screening history:

DOCTOR: What are you allergic to?
YOU: Spring.
DOCTOR: Me too. Here's some allergy medicine, not that I believe in allergies.

You can see why I'm happy I don't have allergies. No, I'm sure what I have is vasomotor rhinitis, a common condition where your nose clogs up and your life is miserable FOR NO PARTICULAR REASON, which is still better than being at the annual mercy of the pollen count.

Of course, pills are not the only treatment, which leads me to say a word about allergy shots: "Ouch." Say, for example, you are allergic to cats. (You find out by getting 300 little scratches on your skin, many of them carrying dust, mold, spores or fungus.) There are really two treatments: 1. Stay away from cats, or 2. You and the cat become blood relatives by having tiny bits of cat hair injected under your skin every week for five years. In some patients this constant exposure uses up all the allergies and helps relieve their stuffy noses, although it can cause troublesome hairballs.

As goofy as this sounds, allergy shots actually help some people, unless they are just saying this to avoid more treatments:

PATIENT: No, I feel better, I swear. Really.
DOCTOR: Let's inject you with some more mold and fungus, just to be on the safe side.

As you can see, allergies are no fun. I'm sure my own spring-time nasal problems are caused by some other condition, perhaps by a slow leaking of cerebrospinal fluid from a tiny crack in my skull where I bumped my head on the garage door last week. This would mean just a matter of time before the rest of the fluid runs out, causing severe brain damage and forcing me into an institution or congressional office.

What a lucky break—at least it's not allergies.

Life and Death Insurance Physicals

For a long time I have been following one of the important rules for living a long, healthy life, which says never get a physical for the purpose of buying insurance.

It hasn't been easy. I am always getting a lot of advice from various financial-type people, often over the phone during dinner. For some reason, they always want me to buy life insurance, although they usually call it something else:

Financial person: This new variable universal comprehensive investment term plan is guaranteed to pay you a net return of not less than $3 million, at a total cost to you of $6.98 plus postage.
Me: What do I have to do?
Financial person: Just take a simple insurance physical.
Me: What? For only $3 million?

Life insurance policies always require a physical exam, unlike health insurance. (Health insurers do not need a comprehensive exam and laboratory testing to turn you down—they often do this over the phone, sometimes with a recorded message.) Basically, the insurance company wants you to prove that you are healthy enough to send them money every month for the rest of your life.

I have always been uneasy with the life insurance concept, probably because I was a student for such a long time. For many years I was worth a lot more dead than alive, which was not something I wanted any of those cutthroat premed students to know. Even later, when I had a job, I still managed to avoid having insurance doctors poking and prodding me with various medical devices in the privacy of my own home.

I have done many of these physicals on other people, and as far as I can tell, an insurance physical can only determine one thing: whether or not you are going to die during the physical. When you buy life insurance you are actually betting a large sum of money that you are going to die sometime soon. The insurance people are betting against it, at least not until they have had a chance to cover the cost of the annual insurance company Christmas party. Not even the federal government could sell a lottery that you win by dying young.

Believe me, doctors don't like these physicals any more than patients do. Instead of asking about important risk factors, insurance companies ask doctors to do goofy things like taking measurements of the person's chest. Every insurance company wants to know this, as if it is going to give you a new suit if you pass the exam.

They also ask us to measure your heart rate after exercise, although they never say what exercise. They may assume you will be running 440-meter hurdles in our lobby, but we usually just have you go up and down on a little step. This is required to weed out the people who are hanging by a thread, cardiac-wise, and who will die from the least bit of strain. Insurance companies would much rather have this happen in the doctor's office, before any forms are signed. I would not be surprised if they started asking us for the heart rate while hang gliding over rapids or deactivating concussion mines.

Even if you make it through the rest, you will still need to provide "the sample." In the old days this meant following strict rules of evidence, and the lab technician had to actually witness you producing "the sample" into a little cup. Not many people can perform for a command audience like that. Fortunately, most doctor's offices now have new, miniaturized technology which allows them to conceal a powerful video camera in what appears to be an ordinary faucet.

"The sample" is then sent to the insurance company through the mail, which should make any young person think twice about a career as a postal inspector.

Finally, the physical is over, your doctor sends in the forms, and you can settle back and relax, knowing you will never hear a word from the company again. After a few months you may want to call, but don't expect them to talk to you. Insurance companies are careful not to give any information about yourself to you directly. They don't want to do anything that might alter your life expectancy, allowing you to collect sooner than they want you to. Because the truth is, it's not really life insurance at all. None of these companies will give you a nickel for staying alive. It's really death insurance— the marketing people changed the name long ago to make it easier to sell at parties and wedding receptions.

That's why I don't get insurance physicals. All they can tell me is that I am going to die someday. That's something I already know too well, even if I don't want to put any money on it.

Lawn Mower Maintenance for Your Body

Most of us can hardly wait for Spring, so we can begin enjoying our favorite sports-related injuries.

This year, before returning to your usual strenuous lifestyle, spend some time checking over your body to make sure it is in good working condition. Although doctors never really explain this process to their patients, these checkups can be done using the handy checklists for routine lawn-mower maintenance that appear in newspapers every spring.

These lists, which are loaded with important maintenance tips, are presented each year by lawn and garden experts to make the rest of us feel guilty. For myself, the closest I ever come to routine lawn-mower care is trying not to hit it with the car while pulling into the garage.

Although never actually used on lawn mowers, many of these points can be adapted to provide effective springtime maintenance for our bodies as well:

• Check the heart and large arteries for poorly fitting connections or leaks. Make sure the heartbeat is strong and smooth, providing a quick-starting and smooth-running pulse, without gaps or skips as you begin to move around off the couch.

• Check the central belt for tightness. If the tension is too high, let it out a few notches, or switch to sweat pants.

• To prime the stomach after a winter of holiday buffets and televised sporting events, pour 2 to 3 tablespoons of fresh Gatorade into the bottom of the stomach housing.

• Inspect the stomach itself. Scrape away any jalapeno bean dip deposits that have accumulated over the winter. These can form a gummy substance that fouls the intestinal tract. To clean, pour in a little caustic, horrible-tasting mouthwash like Listerine, slosh it around and then drain. Fill with fresh whole-grain Wheaties.

• Before each use, check to see that the circulatory system is filled to the recommended level, preferably with the kind of fluid not found in aluminum cans.

• Inspect the vertebral column. If frayed or worn, avoid jumping or twisting activities, or have it replaced altogether.

• Using a hand mirror and a powerful flashlight, inspect the lung filter elements, those tiny little hairs inside the nose. Thoroughly clean any blocked airway passages, vacuuming if necessary. If the lungs remain blocked, wash thoroughly in hot soapy water, rinse, and then gently squeeze out the water. Allow to air dry.

• Following the instructions in the original owner's manual, relubricate the knees, spreading the joint fluid evenly over all surface areas before jogging, running, or even thinking of standing on artificial turf.

• Inspect the feet. If they are badly nicked, or have severe toenail damage, have them realigned by a professional. Removing more than a cuticle yourself will place an uneven load on the legs, causing blisters and poor Nike wear.

• And don't forget to clean the exterior thoroughly after each use, scrubbing gently with mild deodorant soap and a soft rag. Spray penetrating antiperspirant on exposed glands and between other moving parts. This can prevent embarrassing after-burn fumes that would bother people at the ice cream counter afterward.

Ask the Doctor

Judging by my mail, some readers have a lot of questions about recent developments on the medical scene. This is scary, because it means they do not have access to any better source of health care than me. It is just another reason to hope that Hillary Rodham Clinton knows what she is doing.

In the meantime, I will try to provide some answers so some of these people can get back to watching the home shopping network:

Q: I hear there is a new screening test for prostate cancer, but my insurance company won't cover it. Is there a way I can be sure my insurance company gets cancer?

A: Most insurance companies carefully investigate any new screening tests, reviewing all the available clinical research before deciding not to pay for them. They sometimes reevaluate, but only after new research or a sensational story on a show like "A 20/20 Current Inside Affair."

Q: Which is it, "starve a fever," or "starve a cold," or what?

A: The correct saying, "Starve a fever and feed a cold," was derived from the ancient Yiddish, "Feed a fever, or starve it, whatever, I don't care, but never, ever turn your back on a goiter." This was later shortened to the more familiar version, "Feed a fever and starve a cold," which is, of course, the correct saying.

Q: Why don't you ever hear about radon gas anymore?

A: You'd think the radon gas threat was over. You rarely see any more magazine articles like "Radon, the Deadly Creeping Silent Killer Menace From the Earth." Most people can identify "radon" only as the enormous pterodactyl that attacked Tokyo in several Godzilla movies. But according to informed government sources (a helpful woman at the Health Department named "Sheila"), radon is still something to worry about. Some criminals made thousands of dollars in the 1980s selling unlicensed radon detectors, which actually turned positive around certain types of cheese, but you can now get legitimate, EPA-approved radon detectors for $24.95 from the American Lung Association. I'd ask for Sheila.

Q: Is it a good idea to take "Grapefruit Burners," "Megalo Vitamins," or any of the other diet aids shown on late-night TV?

A: It is an excellent idea, as long as you are independently wealthy and don't really expect to lose weight. Remember, diet supplements only work when combined with a good program of regular exercise. I recommend the "Gut Buster," $49.95 after midnight on most channels.

Q: Is there some chemical in the California water supply that causes serious brain damage in television and movie stars, forcing them to parade their personal tragedies in the media and drag themselves and their families through months of public degradation and talk-show humiliation, just to appear on the covers of magazines and newspapers sold only in grocery stores?

A: Yes.

Q: Are there some real diseases that just sound too goofy to diagnose?

A: Yes. For example, newborn babies are no longer routinely tested for "Maple Syrup Urine Disease," mostly because it is very rare and doctors got tired of trying to explain it. And doctors pray that no one will ever come to their office with symptoms of "Blue Rubber Bleb Nevus Syndrome." Nobody would believe them.

Q: A friend told me that a lot of babies are born just before a hurricane hits, because of the low pressure or something. Is this true?

A: Your friend is either a real poodle-brain or a trained medical professional. Medicine is full of myths, and doctors and nurses in coastal areas believed this for years. I suppose they thought the sudden swings in atmospheric pressure just sucked the babies right out. This was disproved during Hurricane Andrew, which was lucky because the emergency rooms were already busy enough, there being a full moon and everything.

Q: Don't you get angry letters from certain plastic surgeons, like the ones whose ads feature women's buttocks, after making fun of things like liposuction?

A: No, those particular plastic surgeons have been surprisingly tolerant for a bunch of pompous, money-grubbing parasites. They have been able to turn aside my gentle, good-natured criticism, knowing deep in their hearts that no one will ever perform cosmetic surgery on me. I am doomed to spend the rest of my life looking like the picture on the front of this book. Apparently, this is punishment enough.

Ask Him Again

It's time again to "Ask The Doctor," the popular feature where I get to pretend I actually provide useful medical information to readers. Doctors love to write these features because it lets them address important medical questions while having readers do half the work for free. Remember, patient confidentiality prevents me from using their names, unless the question is really silly.

Q: How come you never hear about older diseases like scurvy or lumbago any more?

A: In the old days, medicine was much easier. For example, back then "heart" was an actual diagnosis, as in, "Doc says it's my heart." There were only about six different diseases, including "heart," "kidneys," and "the vapors." Anything not on the list was simply called "a spell."

   Now, with medicine progressing at a startling rate, we just don't have room for every disease. Occasionally, some of the older ones get dropped to make room. Not many doctors even know what "lumbago" means any more. Many think it is "a type of trailer home." Thanks to this weeding-out process we have room for modern, up-to-date diseases like agoraphobia, the fear of public places. This disease did not even exist 30 years ago, when everyone just stayed home anyway.

Q: Are home cholesterol tests a good idea?

A: Testing your own cholesterol is now possible, thanks to a new home kit just approved by the FDA. Like other in-home tests, these products, while not terribly accurate, can finally let people know if they have a problem without having to see the doctor. A blue dot on testing means you definitely have a cholesterol problem, or else strep throat, or you might be pregnant. To find out which, you'll have to see a doctor.

Q: Are tanning booths safe?

A: When dealing with ultraviolet radiation, "safe" is a relative term, meaning only that there are no visible burns on your body when you leave. The only signs of tanning booth activity are two white spots where your shoulder blades were in contact with the lead shielding, which makes you look like a large hyena.

Still, we now know that any exposure to sunlight is risky, especially in a hinged, coffin-shaped tanning bed. People assume that tanning booths are strictly regulated, but the only real requirement seems to be some experience in video rental. While owners insist they tightly control the different types of ultraviolet radiation, surveys of these people show that most of them think U.V.A. is a college in Virginia and U.V.B. is a cable TV channel ("All Ultraviolet, All The Time.")

Even Coppertone now recognizes the connection between tanning and death. The cute little girl in their new logo now wears a shirt and big, goofy hat (Experts agree that goofy hats are the best protection.) This is a significant change from their old ads, which featured teenage models wearing swimsuits the size of microbes, slathering themselves in Coppertone Deep Tan Frying Oil, which has an SPF of 0.002, making two minutes on the beach the equivalent of a week on the surface of Mercury. A few years later these same models were appearing as extras in "The Golden Girls," which led the company to make a few changes.

Q: How can you tell if your dog needs Prozac?

A: Chronic barking, according to some veterinarians who now routinely prescribe the medication for their furry patients. Also depression, malaise, and aggressive behavior, although these symptoms might also mean that you are really dealing with a cat. While Prozac may not be able to transform a cat into an actual pet, it can help relieve certain symptoms like tail chasing, which can be bothersome to pet owners who do not want animals having more fun than they do.

Q: You know in the popular movie *Wolf*, where Jack Nicholson goes to the doctor because he is turning into an animal and killing deer with his teeth, and the doctor tells him not to worry, that he was probably just sleepwalking and should go to the hospital for "some tests"? shouldn't that doctor be shot or something?

A: Yes. Doctors in monster movies are always incredible idiots. They act like they don't even realize they are in a movie. Most of the time they are soon torn to shreds by the monster, sparing them the even worse horror of a malpractice suit.

Q: How do dermatologists treat moles?

A: Just like anyone else, according to a dermatologist friend of mine, who recommends flooding their little tunnels with a hose while setting live traps around the garden. As far as SKIN moles, the only new development is that some people are now going to dermatologists to have moles put on. Evidently, they think doctors who remove moles have been saving them for later transplantation onto anyone wanting to look like Cindy Crawford. Obviously, people like this require specialized treatment. I recommend live traps.

Q: Can doctors be funny?

A: No. A medical exam room is no place for comedy. Laughing during a doctor's appointment is considered "abnormal," and the Hippocratic oath requires the doctor to send these people for immediate psychiatric counseling.

Instead, some doctors write books. This satisfies their need for humorous expression and generates a lot of mail, giving them plenty of reasons to get counseling themselves.

Let's Get Physicals

Summer vacation means swimming, bike riding, playing baseball, and just generally goofing off. It is also time for school physicals, which means that doctors have to stop doing all those things and get back to the office.

Any doctors who take care of children are busy every summer doing school physicals. They start off in June doing one or two a day, a number which gradually increases until the last day before school starts, when they have to do about 3,000 for all the parents who forgot to make appointments.

The main reason for these check-ups is to make sure all children get the proper immunizations, which are important to keep them healthy. These days there are so many different shots (DPT, MMR, HIB, HEP-B, IRS, GATT, etc.) that parents can not possibly keep track, so the schools periodically send them to doctors, who remember to write them down.

This process begins with "Kindergarten Round-up," an annual summer event where new students and their parents can mosey on down to the old school house to rustle up a mess o' forms for the doc to sign before starting school. The children are rounded up, weighed, measured, and branded with school name and grade level, like "Lazy Bar-K, p.m. bus." (They don't really use a branding iron—it's more like an indelible marker.)

Next the parents bring all of the forms to the doctor's office, where nurses check their vision, hearing, ambient temperature, tensile strength, and several other technical specifications, putting check marks in the little boxes on the forms.

After that, it's time to see the doctor. I enjoy these preschool visits, and not just because the nurses do most of the work. Physicals like this are very important to determine if five year-old children, who have been in constant motion since birth, are healthy enough to sit still in a classroom for four hours a day. Most of them pass easily. All the doctor has to do is check their ears and play with the Power Ranger action figures they brought with them.

Children enjoy these visits, too. At this stage they are looking forward to school, ready to enter an exciting world of promise and adventure, while still feeling safe and protected in the arms of their parents. Then we give them a shot.

Actually, the nurse gives the shot. I try to be out of the room at the time, coming back with a sticker after the crying is over.

The other popular time for school physicals is at age 12, just before junior high. These physicals are important to determine if the budding teen is healthy enough to wear enormous pants and listen to music groups with names like "Hemorrhaging Death Weasels."

I enjoy these visits too. It's my job to warn these older children about the things that make life a scary place, like smoking, drinking, and unsafe sex. I also try to encourage them in sports and other healthy activities, although by this time many of them have been playing sports long enough to have their uniform numbers retired. Organized hockey, for example, now begins in utero, requiring parents to purchase several full sets of equipment even before birth.

At twelve, the differences between girls and boys are just becoming obvious. For example, girls often arrive with their mothers, with whom they actively converse. Some are animated and excited, talking over plans for the coming school year and sharing their innermost dreams and aspirations for the future. So we give them a shot.

Boys may also come with their mothers, but within seconds they are begging them to leave and wait in the lobby. The average 12 year-old boy would sooner be examined on public access cable TV than to have his own mother in the room. Mothers are sometimes shocked by this request, especially when they have not heard their sons speak in several years.

The boys prefer it this way because it allows them to have their impending panic attack in private. For some reason, teen age boys love to tease each other about going to the doctor. By the time they get to the office they are experiencing heart palpitations from worrying about 1) the shot, and 2) the hernia check. They are convinced that the doctor is going to use a whaling harpoon for one and a pneumatic locking vise-grips for the other.

It is up to the doctor to calm them down, showing them that a simple medical exam is not painful and should be nothing to worry about. Then we give them a shot.

They can then go back to the lobby, where they resume not talking to their parents until many years later, when they need money for college. At that point they will usually need another physical, which is very important to find out if they are healthy enough to stay up nights drinking coffee and going to law school. I enjoy those visits. Sometimes I even choose to give the shots myself.

Breakthroughs & Breakdowns

Medical research is advancing at an amazing rate. Every month the medical journals are full of reports like, "Blond, fair-skinned left-handed pipe welders shown more susceptible to gall bladder disease."

Aside from the obvious questions (How does this help anyone? What are they supposed to do, dye their hair?), you have to wonder who is coming up with these research topics, and, more important, whether they should be forced to find real jobs.

The Year They Saved Smallpox

Every year seems filled with many remarkable events that have shaped the field of medicine. Unfortunately, none of us can remember them without those "year in review" articles that appear every December. Here are some amazing events that took place in just one year:

• A scientist in Georgia has been collecting spit samples from men in hopes of learning why they are such jerks. Dr. James Dabbs, a psychologist at Georgia State, believes that higher levels of testosterone may be present in the saliva of aggressive and antisocial men, like the ones who put their samples directly on his shoes instead of in the collecting jar. His results could shed new light on the behavior of criminals and professional baseball players, who spit for a living.

• *Jurassic Park,* a movie about the dangers of cloning dinosaurs, became the top-grossing movie of all time. It triggered a long string of articles by scientific experts, stating that cloning dinosaurs, as depicted in the movie, is impossible and could never be accomplished. Meanwhile, other scientists were busy creating clones of human embryos, just to prove they could. These cloned human embryos were also the subject of an intense debate, as psychologists everywhere warned parents not to take their children to see them.

• Despite sensational news reports and several lawsuits, it was finally shown that cellular telephones do not cause brain cancer. According to research, those people driving with one hand while talking into car phones do not really have brain damage. They only drive that way.

• As part of the ongoing effort to make science more exciting, researchers discovered the specific chemical responsible for triggering penile erections. By stimulating rats with electrodes, scientists were able to check their blood levels and determine that nitric oxide caused erections in the males, at least the really twisted ones. Although this experiment seems cruel, it was more acceptable than their original plan of taking blood from male junior high students who had just been sent to the blackboard. Scientists say the discovery will have direct clinical applications within five years, or if nothing else will be good for a few laughs at parties.

• Between health reform and malpractice suits, physicians have received a lot of bad press in the last few years. Doctors everywhere were glad when the media decided to select one physician and give him extensive, in-depth coverage throughout the year, chronicling his dedication and commitment, and letting everyone appreciate the results of his tireless work with patients. Unfortunately, the doctor they picked was Jack Kevorkian.

• Although smallpox was eradicated back in 1977, a few hundred specimens of the deadly virus have been kept frozen in Atlanta and Moscow. Scientists were scheduled to destroy them, subjecting the virus to death by boiling and totally wiping out smallpox, but a last minute outcry made them put their plans on hold. Evidently, there are some scientists who feel that smallpox should be rehabilitated, believing that it's not a bad virus, just misunderstood. Now those lethal specimens are back in cold storage, costing thousands of dollars and taking up valuable freezer space that could otherwise be used for cloned dinosaur embryos.

• Cardiologists discovered that men with bald spots had an increased risk of heart attacks. Although the news sent men running to the Hair Club, the actual increased risk was less than the risk of smoking or going without exercise. Both baldness and heart disease are thought to be direct effects of the male hormone testosterone. This is more evidence that males will be disappearing from the planet altogether as soon as women find a way to reproduce without them (see "nitric oxide," above).

• And finally, medical science made another tremendous leap backward, releasing new evidence that drinking alcohol daily can help protect you from heart disease. This follows the 1992 discovery that very low cholesterol levels can also be bad for you, leading to a higher chance of dying from other causes, particularly murder. While some of these deaths were undoubtedly provoked by bragging, the headlines blamed low cholesterol. This resulted in a tremendous jump in Hostess Twinkie sales nationwide.

Now a new study may do the same for alcohol. New research shows that moderate drinking can protect you from heart disease. Because of this, many people will be waving tattered copies of this book the next time they go to a bar in an attempt to lower both their heart risk and I.Q.

This is just another good reason to stay home. Stay away from electrodes, boil up any viruses you have around the house, and try to stay healthy. After all, you never know what's in store for us next year.

Estrogen Memories

A recent research study shows that estrogen may prevent memory loss in Alzheimer's patients. This must have been startling news to anyone from the planet Zorg, but really, the rest of us should have been able to figure it out.

The study shows that women taking estrogen for hot flashes or osteoporosis were 40 percent less likely to develop Alzheimer's, a neurological disorder that causes severe, disabling memory loss. While most people don't have Alzheimer's, it is something that folks over 30 think about every time they misplace their car keys. We all experience various degrees of memory loss throughout our lifetimes. Our brain cells begin dying off around the time we start memorizing the multiplication tables in grade school, and the process accelerates after algebra and calculus.

Now it seems that estrogen may protect those brain cells. Researchers believe that the female hormone may help preserve normal memory function in certain areas of the mind. According to one expert, "Estrogen is a very important hormone for the brain."

At least for some brains. Men, as a rule, have little or no estrogen in their heads, which says a lot about why they have trouble remembering certain details like anniversaries or the names of first-degree relatives. Men are generally exposed to estrogen only through contact with women. The only effect of that estrogen on the male brain is to cause it to shut down, leaving men to think with other, less intelligent parts of their anatomy.

This new estrogen theory is much better than other attempts to explain this problem. For a long time scientists believed that there was a chemical imbalance in some male brains that was triggered by marriage, possibly by something in wedding cake. Studies showed that even competent, professional males were sometimes turned into helpless amnesia victims after marriage, becoming suddenly unable to remember phone numbers, birthdays or exactly where to put their clean socks. For some men, the last important date they ever remembered was their wedding day. Once they made it to the ceremony, their wives took over. It now seems clear that this is not merely a result of brain damage in men, but is due to estrogen deficiency.

Thanks to their hormones, women have built-in protection against this kind of memory problem. As a male, my reaction is: What? Again?? Estrogen already protects women from heart disease, making them 50 percent less likely to have heart attacks. Just being a male is as much of a cardiac risk factor as diabetes, smoking, or having a "frequent diner" card at Old Country Buffet. Any man over 50 automatically has two strikes against him when it comes to heart disease, but women have estrogen to protect them. All they lose in return is the ability to enjoy James Bond movies and an affinity for tossing things around inside the house.

News like this would certainly make estrogen pills even more popular, if only that were possible. Premarin, the most common brand-name estrogen, is already the second-most prescribed medicine in the country, with some doctors believing that every woman should take it for life. After this news they might as well start putting it in Diet Coke.

Unfortunately, the research study did not answer the question of whether estrogen can protect memory in anyone, not just women. If future studies can show a similar benefit, men everywhere may someday have to decide if the ability to remember details is worth a few small changes in appearance, like losing facial hair and growing breasts.

Until then, medical science has come up with some very reassuring news for half of the population. If you are a woman, you can rest easy, knowing your hormones are working overtime to protect you from another disease threat.

And if you are a man, don't worry—you'll never remember reading this anyway.

Keep an Ear on Reattachment

There have been a lot of reattachment stories in the news lately, and this has me thinking a little differently about my limbs.

For example, John Thompson is a young man from North Dakota whose arms were severed above the elbow by a harvesting machine. Through determination and some unbelievable force of will, John managed to get himself back to the house and call for help.

Those arms are now a part of him again, thanks to incredible reattachment surgery. When last seen on TV, John was smiling and waving with one of those arms, now firmly back on his shoulder where it belongs.

Michael Conoboy was not quite so lucky. After he was injured, again by farm machinery, doctors were able to save only one of his arms. Still, at last report it was back in place and doing well.

Cases like these still seem like miracles. New technology allows doctors to use high-powered microscopes and instruments the size of an ant's jaws to reconnect individual nerves and arteries, making these incredible results possible. You can bet that we will be hearing about even more amazing cases in the future.

In fact, earlier this year I learned about another successful reattachment procedure. I was listening to my car radio at the time, as I often am when I learn about amazing medical breakthroughs.

What I heard was very exciting, and I wanted to take down some of the details. Unfortunately, I was almost killed while trying to pull to the side of the road, but I did manage to scribble some notes onto the back of a Taco Bell bag that we keep in the car for emergencies like this. I knew it would be worth it, if only to convince the people who think that I make up these things.

The story took place in a London hospital. A patient was taken there after a fight in a pub, with one severed ear packed in ice. (As a medical professional, I am not able to reveal his name, even though the radio did. Besides, a small blotch of taco sauce made that part of my notes unreadable.) According to reports, the ear was bitten off in the fight, leaving it much too mangled and bruised to allow simple reattachment.

Luckily, a Royal Professor of Plastic Surgery was handy, and after several hours of intense operating he was able to reimplant the damaged ear tissue, although in a spot about 2 1/2 feet (or 0.67 meters, since we're talking about England) lower than its original position. The ear ended up attached to the inner thigh of the patient, near the large blood vessels that run through the groin.

That's correct: The surgeon reattached the ear, on purpose, to the patient's thigh.

According to the plastic surgeon, he needed to put the ear where there was a better blood supply. He planned on transferring it back to the head after four or five months, when the healing was complete.

At the risk of permanently damaging some vital humor reflex, I am refraining from making any easy "ear-groin" jokes here. I will say one thing: I wish I had been in the room when he explained his plan to the patient. I assume he asked for permission first, although it's hard to imagine that anyone would agree to have something reattached to their head that had been spending the last five months in his groin.

They did interview the surgeon, although I am not able to give you his name (bean burrito smear). While he made no mention of the patient's reaction, he did describe some of his other cases in this exciting field. "Microvascular reattachment is the next frontier," he said. "Two years ago we did the same thing with a severed hand from a traffic accident. We implanted it on the chest wall, right below the left nipple. After four months we moved it back, and the patient eventually regained some use of the hand."

I tried to concentrate, despite the mental picture I was forming of this procedure. The surgeon went on to make some bold predictions for the future.

"It will be a time," he said, "when we will all be able to replace our body parts with newer, more attractive pieces." He said this like it was somehow different from what plastic surgeons have been doing in this country for years, but by this time I had pulled back into traffic and was driving away.

Obviously, if doctors are making this kind of progress with arms and ears, it is just a matter of time until all of our parts become expendable. Someday the FDA may be asked to regulate implants for other replacement body parts, although its record in this area leaves a lot to be desired.

Until then, I am going to play it safe. I'll be more careful driving my car, and I think I'll just stay away from farm machinery altogether.

Magnet Heads and Bird Brains

A lot of people were surprised by new medical research that proves we all have tiny little magnets in our brains. Not me. I think it explains a lot.

It was a team of researchers at the California Institute of Technology who discovered that there are microscopic crystals called "magnetite" scattered throughout human brain tissue.

The reason this is important, in case you were wondering, is that these magnetized particles may be the same ones that other species of animals use to accurately navigate over long distances.

Scientists already knew that these particles are present in certain types of birds. They believe that they may explain their uncanny sense of direction, besides shedding some light on some of their other, more oddball behavior.

For one thing, the magnet theory might explain why the woodpeckers in my neighborhood are always attacking our metal chimney. You can hear them up there, usually around 5:30 A.M., making a noise like a garbage can in a hailstorm. I have never understood what they were after—as far as I can tell, there are no insects in sheet metal, and I can't believe they want to build a nest in a chimney (the fire insurance premiums would be staggering.) Modern magnet theory, however, tells us that they just can't help themselves.

It also explains their little problem with windows. Here is a species with advanced navigation technology, and somehow they still regularly manage to fly right smack into the middle of our picture window. From my desk I can see one of them out there right now, sitting on the grass and rubbing his little bird head as he tries to figure out what went wrong. The answer is obvious: glass is non-magnetic; it doesn't register on their magnetite. Now, thanks to research, I know that all I have to do is cover the window with aluminum foil and the problem is solved.

If nothing else, it is another good reason, as if anybody needed another one, not to keep those large, evil-looking carnivorous birds in your home as pets. You know the ones I mean—the ones with the curving, hook-like beaks designed for ripping flesh from bones. Sure, they're colorful, and they can simulate human speech (often to lure children toward their cages,) but once in your house their brain magnetism could set up some kind of interference pattern with your own. Soon you would start thinking strange, birdlike thoughts, and then one day the police would find you down at the playground, perched on the jungle gym and waiting for Tippi Hedren to pass by.

You can see why this new magnetism research is important: Now we know that magnetism affects human behavior as well as bird brains. Remember that kid at summer camp who could always find his way back to the tent, no matter how deep in the woods you left him behind? Everyone always said he had a good sense of direction. Evidently, what he had was a good set of magnets.

Everyone knows some people attract others, while some, most notably attorneys, tend to repel. Now there is scientific evidence that this is just simple physics. It is magnetism that makes our heads spin around like little black-and-white Scottie dogs when an attractive person walks by, just as it catapults us out of the room when an insurance salesman opens his briefcase.

This would also account for the way that some people are affected by overhead power lines. There are several high-voltage lines above the hospital parking lot where I work, and the current in those babies is enough to create a humming noise like a blender on "puree." I'm sure they carry enough electromagnetic charge to mess with my magnetite. Several times I have found myself driving my car in circles underneath the wires, trying to remember how to get home.

And of course, now we can finally understand why it is so hard to walk past a refrigerator without stopping. And why some people can hang spoons from their noses.

Once again, medical research has made a real difference in our lives. The magnet study shows that we are creatures of simple polarity. If nothing else, it may finally answer the question that people in other parts of the country have been asking for years, especially during network news reports that show us tunneling through snowdrifts to our cars: Why would anyone want to live in Minnesota, so close to the north pole?

Research tells us that, like the birds, we may have little choice.

Crazy for Prozac

It would be crazy to ignore a recent study in the American Psychiatric Journal showing that 50 percent of all Americans will experience mental illness at some time during their lives. This seems like a pretty high number until you consider what they mean by "illness." Most people think mental illness means truly dysfunctional behavior, like pulling the wings off full-grown birds or following orders from tiny gnomes living in your ear canals. This study, however, took a much broader view, even including people who continually lose their car keys or who scream at the TV during sporting events.

This is because the research was done by psychiatrists, who are trained to look for mental illness. Some of them can even detect thought disturbances in inanimate objects. During residency they practice by analyzing medical students, giving them a skewed notion of how common these problems are.

This study is significant because doctors have gotten much better at treating some of these borderline problems. If someone gives you a hammer, you start to notice a lot of loose nails, and in the last few years doctors have been handed the therapeutic equivalent of a Craftsman model 2000 pneumatic power nailer.

Its name is Prozac, and you already know someone who takes it. You may even take it yourself. (If you aren't sure, it could mean one of your other personalities has been going to the doctor without you.)

Originally used for treating depression, Prozac has become one of the top-selling prescription medicines in history, and as common as Amoxicillin in a day care center.

It is frightening how fast Prozac exploded onto the popular scene. Without advertising directly to patients (yet), the name

"Prozac" has become as recognizable as "Coca-Cola." Friends compare prescription bottles, radio announcers tease each other about forgetting their morning doses, and people talk about "Prozac moments" the way they used to talk about "Excedrin headaches." It's become so popular, in fact, that it even turns up on TV. Most stand-up comics can do 10 minutes on Prozac. The medicine is routinely featured in late-night monologues and even on sitcoms, where obnoxious child actors can talk freely about psychiatric medicines as long as they don't mention condoms.

All of this has changed the way doctors diagnose depression.

People with this disease used to come to the doctor complaining of feeling tired. It often took several visits and a special questionnaire to show they were actually depressed, and another few visits to decide if medication might help.

Now they come in saying, "I want Prozac." The whole visit, diagnosis to prescription, takes about three minutes. They already feel better when they leave.

Doctors can do this because Prozac is very safe, and because its beneficial effects go way beyond just depression. It seems to help a variety of other conditions as well, from obsessive-compulsive disorder to Claustrophobia, the unreasoning fear of Santa.

Some psychiatrists now prescribe it for "dysthymia," a kind of depression "lite" that can apply to anyone not currently laughing. There is evidence that Prozac improves all functions of the brain, even the ones that keep track of the car keys.

All of which is turning Prozac into a household name. It's hard to imagine this kind of response to, say, a new antifungal cream, but the fame of Prozac continues to spread. Several other drug companies have picked up on the trend, releasing new, improved versions of Prozac that offer such important therapeutic advantages as designer colors or pills that are lighter and easier to lift to your mouth. As the competition heats up we'll undoubtedly see more direct ads, with TV and radio commercials, billboards, and, of course, celebrity endorsements.

As with anything so popular, the backlash has already begun. Newsweek ran an alarming cover story about the dangers of "designing personalities." In "Listening to Prozac," the bestselling psychiatry textbook ever, Dr. Jeffrey Kramer wonders if tinkering with brain chemistry is really a good idea, even though as a psychiatrist he continues to do it on a daily basis. News stories warn us of an army of mindless Prozac zombies, who smile at you and say "thanks" when you run over their feet on the curb.

Maybe, but major depression is some scary stuff. While it's hard to believe that so many people need help with their brain chemistry, it's also hard to predict who might be helped, or even saved, by medicine.

At least the popularity of Prozac brought the subject of depression out into the open. It may not be for everyone, but, thanks to publicity, people everywhere (and their doctors) are now more aware of the problem. This is just another example of doctors learning from Jay Leno.

Personally, I'm glad. You never know when your half of the population will be coming up.

Blood Researchers Go Hog Wild

I've been feeling quite a sense of relief these days, what with the fall of communism in Eastern Europe, the end of the Gulf War, and mutant pigs that produce human blood.

I know, it sounds like I made it up, but it is absolutely true: Communism in Europe is pretty much dead.

The part about the pigs is also true, at least according to a recent New York Times article, "Mutated pigs producing human hemoglobin." It explains that a bunch of scientists in New Jersey have injected human genes into pigs, teaching them to make human hemoglobin. What it doesn't say is how they came up with the idea in the first place.

I like to imagine a bunch of researchers at happy hour, sitting around a table saying things like, "Wait, what about this one? We get some human genes and we inject them—into PIGS! Get it? Isn't that great?"

Evidently, the bloodmaking cells in these piglets use the genes as tiny recipe cards, turning part of their blood into human-type blood. None of the scientists was willing to come right out and say this was in any way an improvement over your average pig, but the implication was clear.

The article was obviously meant to be reassuring. "Go ahead,"it says, "Bleed all you want. We'll make more." I think this kind of breakthrough is encouraging, although I hope readers don't get the wrong idea. I hate to think of anyone seeing the "mutant pig" story and then deciding to open a porcupine ranch, or to take up a dangerous hobby like juggling chain saws. Certainly, it would be wonderful to have a safe blood supply, although in this day and age I am sure even pigs will have to answer a few questions about their health habits and sexual preferences.

But the article goes even a step further: It says the pig blood will "offer advantages over the donated blood now being used," that donated blood presumably coming largely from humans. I guess we have finally reached the point where people can no longer be trusted to do important things like make their own blood. For safety reasons, we are better off leaving it to pigs.

I still have a lot of questions, though. What kind of side effects will there be? I'm already kind of messy around the house. What would I be like after a transfusion of swine "O" positive? Will recipients of the new hemoglobin start spending their warm summer afternoons down at the neighborhood slough? Will mud wrestling become the great American pastime?

What if people decide to forget about blood banks altogether? They may figure they can use their own pigs, in the privacy of their own sty. People in Beverly Hills will rely on their own cute little pot-bellied hogs, finally giving them a legitimate reason to keep those things as pets.

Of course, pigs are supposed to be very smart animals. I'm sure that's why they picked them for this important research. But would any pig work? What about guinea pigs? Wart hogs? What about other household pets? My dog is pretty smart—she knows where we keep the doggy treats, and she can "shake" if there's an audience and the mood strikes her. But producing human hemoglobin?

She's probably too old anyway. The scientists started teaching their pigs at one day old. Everyone knows that's too young for dog training, but evidently pigs are ready for chemistry lessons as soon as they open their eyes.

This technology is still experimental, but imagine what will happen when the major drug companies get involved. Some marketing people are going crazy right now trying to think of a name that doesn't sound ridiculous ("Hemo-swine? Plasma-boar? No, I've got it, Pork-u-globin!")

Thank goodness Congress is trying to put a lid on their promotional spending before doctors get flooded by little pig-shaped paper clips and refrigerator magnets.

Well, if the new blood helps save lives, I am all for it. "Experts" were quoted in the article (Medical experts? Farm animal experts?) They called the pig study "a milestone in the effort to find a substitute for human blood."

That's sure comforting news, although for now I think I'll just hang on to the real thing.

Low Cholesterol Eggs

A company in Minnesota has finally broken out its long-awaited new product, the reduced-cholesterol egg.

Like a lot of people, I've known about this new product for a while now. The medical and business pages have been closely following the story of the trendy new eggs as their release date came closer. Brokers and financial planners have also been sending out a lot of information about the new egg technology, hoping to attract a bunch of investors before stock in the company takes off.

"The rollout of the new product will trigger a value-added portfolio of dividend stock options and bond transfers, leading to a fourth quarter dropped percentage on flat revenues, with earning estimates flummoxing the apogee of growth curves by mid-procurement phase. . . ."

This is the reason I'm not a millionaire. I have no idea what these things mean. I get these reports in the mail, and I just throw them away, putting my money in the bank instead like my grandmother always told me to. Because of this, when the stock goes through the roof I'll be standing a safe distance away, where I won't be hit by any flying shingles.

Still, even if I had the money and knew what to do with it, I'm not sure that I would put any of my own eggs in the low-cholesterol basket.

For one thing, they haven't quite worked out the bugs yet. The process, developed by a German company, uses a chemical that binds to the yolk of the egg. The eggs are cracked open and sprayed with the chemical, which is then removed, pulling out most of the cholesterol before it can get into the omelette. Unfortunately, this means that the low-cholesterol eggs will have to be in liquid form.

People have done things like this to eggs before, trying all kinds

57

of ways to get rid of the cholesterol. Unfortunately, all they have managed to come up with are small cartons of "egg substitutes," essentially runny egg whites dyed yellow that taste, well, yellow.

To me, it makes more sense to go right to the source. Up until now, no one has worked on the chickens.

Instead of waiting until the eggs are already laid, why not put the chickens on a comprehensive program of low-fat diet and weight control? This would encourage them to produce leaner and healthier eggs, without any chemicals at all. Farmers could stock up on "Lite 'n Lively" chicken feed, and they could bus the birds to health clubs to work out and watch Cher videos. Their eggs would have to be lower in cholesterol, besides being skinnier and easier to lay.

Of course, this goes against every principle of modern, steroid-enhanced farm theory, but the people have spoken. Their doctors are after them to eat less cholesterol, and they are desperate for the next step in egg evolution. They want healthy, low-cholesterol eggs to eat with their bacon on Saturday mornings, along with slabs of buttered toast and stacks of flapjacks. Eggs are the classic American breakfast food, and people are willing to pay plenty to keep eating them, making a whole bunch of smart investors rich in the process.

And none of them will be me.

Still, I won't be bitter. I have a feeling that whatever egg will be left on my face will still be a far cry from a real one. Technology, although it's pretty good, is not perfect.

Besides, the real problem is the packaging. There are some things that science cannot duplicate, and that includes that perfect wonder of nature called the shell. Until somebody figures out a way to get the new, low-cholesterol eggs back into their original package, I am afraid they will just be another flash in the pan.

Medical Mystery Tour

Like everyone, I was amazed when figure skater Tonya Harding was taken to an emergency room after she was allegedly attacked, only to have the doctors helping her suddenly overwhelmed by noxious fumes emitted from her body. Or am I just confusing two unbelievable, wildly improbable events?

The one about the fumes seems more likely. In this extremely weird and spooky story, a woman in California was brought to the emergency room in cardiac arrest. Sadly, she died, but not before several doctors and nurses were overcome by an unusual chemical odor, winding up in the hospital themselves. Medical people generally have strong stomachs, but this was no ordinary smell. Witnesses say it smelled like organophosphates, the deadly chemicals used to make nerve gas and Shell No-Pest strips, and that it was clearly coming from the woman's body itself. Some of the details are even stranger. Witnesses said her skin had an oily sheen, and one of them saw "white and yellow flecks" in her blood.

I have mixed feelings about medical mysteries like this. Part of me, the scientist part, knows that the autopsy report will eventually give a very reasonable explanation for the problem, blaming some unusual chemical reaction between a particular laundry detergent and the salad dressing she had at her last meal.

Still, until then another part of me will be twitching nervously and saying, "Uh, oh—probably giant parasitic mind-sucking worms from Venus." This is not just because I was the kind of medical student who got into trouble for keeping comic books hidden in his physiology text. It's because I realize that medicine doesn't know everything.

In any science there are things that the experts just haven't figured out yet. Unless you are studying geography, which has been pretty well nailed down by now, there are going to be some unexplained areas that aren't covered in the textbook. This comes up all the time in medicine. At least once a day I tell somebody, "I don't know." Luckily, it's rarely about a serious problem. Often they've just asked a question about that unusual sensation they get in their armpits when they eat Bing cherries, or the click they feel in their elbow while lifting the cat off the VCR. No one has ever asked me why they seem to be emitting nerve gas, causing their family and friends to lose consciousness, but I know what I would say.

This is a scary idea to people who like to believe that doctors know everything about life, the universe and why they are losing their hair, but not me. If nothing else, it takes some of the pressure off doctors, who have been known to torture themselves for forgetting the biochemical structure of ear wax.

Besides, mysteries are exciting. They remind me of the reason I went into medicine in the first place. As a medical student I even got goose bumps from looking inside someone's ear. These days, with Postitron Emission Tomography scans showing us what human thoughts look like while still in the brain, it takes a weird story like mystery nerve gas fumes or spontaneous human combustion to get the feeling back again.

So far, this case has done the job. Even weeks later doctors had no idea why this happened. They performed the autopsy while wearing enough breathing equipment for a deep-sea expedition with Jacques Cousteau, but so far they have no real answers. They are hoping the blood tests will clear things up, but I wouldn't hold my breath.

In the end, they may be forced to do what doctors have always done, assigning the incident a name like "Post-mortem Un-odoriferous (P.U.) Syndrome." They still won't know what happened, but at least they'll be able to write questions for pathology board exams.

Meanwhile, the rest of us will have to wait patiently for an answer, while trying to convince ourselves that this is just an unusual biochemical glitch in the human machinery and not really the first wave of an alien invasion from space. Either way, we probably won't find out until it is too late—and by this I mean until after they make the TV movie.

They have already announced that the story will be used for an episode of the sci-fi program "The X-Files." Being television, the details will be subtly embellished, becoming the story of a beautiful, sexually abused policewoman who develops a mild odor problem after going undercover as a fashion model, but who is saved when doctors discover the problem before terrorists take away her baby. (Based on a true story.)

I know the perfect big-name celebrity to play the woman, unless of course she's back on ice by then.

Bo Knows Hip Surgery

The sports page case report, "Bo Jackson slides on artificial hip," is certainly encouraging news for the budding field of professional athlete reconstruction.

For those not following the Jackson case since his hip replacement, the progress can be summed up through headlines on the sports pages. Ever since training camp after surgery, Bo has made no move without full media coverage. "Bo again in uniform" proved that he could once again put on stretch pants, presumably one leg at a time. "Bo takes batting practice" let us know he could swing a bat, and "Bo steps up to the plate" told us he could still strike out.

If this all seems trivial, remember that this may be the first time an athlete with a prosthesis has been able to compete in any professional sport, unless you count dentures in hockey players.

More than 100,000 hip replacements were performed in this country last year. Not many of those people are making the sports pages. In fact, most of them have to be pretty careful, especially during the months after surgery. Even flexing their leg more than 90 degrees, like sitting on a low chair or toilet seat, might cause the new hip to dislocate. Many of them are eventually able to return to sports like swimming or bicycling, although sports involving jumping, twisting, heavy lifting or body contact are out. Some doctors even discourage walking more than a mile a day, which can make the joint wear out too soon.

What are these people supposed to make of Bo Jackson? They have to wonder if maybe "Bo knows hips" better than their doctors. Soon everyone will be asking for the same artificial hip that was used in Bo, maybe even the Bo Jackson "Autograph" model. With the current trend toward medical advertising, it won't be long before Bo is back on TV with a new set of ads for his own line of prosthetic parts in neon colors, probably made by Nike (new slogan: Just Re-Do It).

The real question is why he would return. As the greatest athlete ever to come out of college, Bo showed good sense in opting for baseball over football, knowing it would keep him healthy in the long run. Unfortunately, this turned out to be a negotiating ploy. Within a year he was playing for the Los Angeles Raiders, injuring his hip and proving his original instinct was a good one.

Now, when the constant abuse of competitive sports might turn his new hip into a rattling peanut in a shell, why take the risk? Even successful replacement parts will wear out soon enough. Anyone younger than 50 can expect to undergo surgery again sometime, even with normal wear and tear on the hip. Sliding into home plate on your bad leg makes for a close play, but it might also mean two canes and a walker later. Bo could stay retired, enjoying life and even playing a little ball with his kids, while living on shoe royalties forever. Why risk it?

We may never know. All we can do is watch the news, waiting for the next headline. And who knows what can happen? "Bo's grand slam wins Series," or maybe "Bo back in football, this time as place kicker." The man has already overcome tremendous odds. Why not again? "Bo takes Belmont, first human to win Triple Crown."

Let's just hope we don't see the other headline instead, the sad one that will prove Bo should have known better.

The Cellulite Scale

Lately I have been trying to come up with a revolutionary idea for a useless new medical product, like the ones you see in health magazines or on late-night TV.

Many fantastic new products like this are invented each year. Most of them are first reported in the back of magazines that also list important developments in the latest soap opera plots. A few become very popular, making it to TV talk shows, and, with a little luck, into Sunday circulars for major department stores.

These products generally make a few simple claims that are very hard to disprove, like promising to completely eradicate every known disease from your body, or extend your natural life span. They are almost always based on the secret discoveries of some ancient civilization whose members are now all dead, making them extremely difficult to sue.

One product like this was invented by a man known as "the Juiceman," who thought up a revolutionary new idea for preparing food, namely grinding it into paste and squeezing the juice out of it. Somehow he was able to convince people that the juice was much better for you than the actual food itself. In fact, through demanding and scrupulous research done in his own kitchen, he was able to come up with a long list of medical problems that could be cured by drinking various combinations of vegetable juices from his machines.

The Juicemaster became a hot item. There were full-page ads in the newspapers, and the Juiceman himself became a health guru, showing up on talk shows everywhere to explain how the "Power of Juicing" could make anyone healthy and slender. Department stores were knee-deep in Juicemasters, Juicemaster Jr.'s, official Juicemaster cookbooks, aprons, glasses and Juicemaster pitchers, along with Juiceman video and audio tapes, featuring the sound of food being ground up. In fact, without these ads the Juicemaster would have been available only from a grandstand booth at State Fairs, and the Juiceman would have been just another huckster with a neck microphone and a slanted mirror over his head.

On the whole, the Juicemaster was pretty successful, rating about an "8" on the Cellulite scale of worthless medical products.This scale ranges from swine flu shots (a "1" on the scale), to the "Thighmaster," which rated a "9" based solely on the number of people staying up late to watch Suzanne Sommers ads on TV. Cellulite is itself a "10" on the scale, being an example of the ideal medical scam. For years, women have been buying creams and lotions to get rid of cellulite. Two or three new products come out every year, from companies with French-sounding names like "La Prarie" (literally, "the prairie") and "Lancombe" ("the comb"). These "anti-cellulite complex" creams are said to have "unique thermo-action" that "helps promote micro-circulation in the skin."

None of which addresses the basic truth about cellulite, which is that it doesn't exist. It is only a scientific-sounding word someone thought up to describe the dimpling effect when extra fat is deposited between the layers of the skin, like adding extra stuffing to an old mattress.

Over the years there has been some serious clinical research into the cellulite question, and the experts all agree. "Just plain garbage," said one noted dermatologist. "There isn't one shred of scientific evidence that these things do any good at all."

The same thing applies to claims made by the Juiceman. In fact, Juicemasters are good for only one thing: making juice. There's nothing wrong with juice, although you would be better off eating your vegetables whole, fiber and all. Just don't expect it to control your blood pressure or fix your fallen arches. Of course, by now most of those Juicemasters are sitting on the top shelves of closets everywhere, next to the pasta machines and hand-held ice cream makers. In fact, this may be the perfect time for me to bring out my revolutionary new concept in health products: the "Wax Maximizer," the New Thermo-Emulsifying Anti-Complex Ear Wax Rejuvenator.

Most people don't realize that the secrets of vitality and long life are contained in ear wax, as discovered by the ancient Abyssinians. Now, thanks to extensive research performed on a few of my close friends and their household pets, the unique health and restorative benefits of ear wax can be yours. In fact, for a limited time, you will also receive the official "Power of Waxing" video, along with a calibrated cerumen scoop autographed by "Dr. Wax" himself.

Act now. After all, the State Fair could be months away.

Low Fat Twinkies

It's hard to know how to react when your world goes topsy-turvy, things stop making sense, and everything you once believed turns out to be a lie. This happened to me when I found out about Hostess Lights Low Fat Twinkies.

For me, this was like dropping a pencil and watching it fall up. There have been a lot of formerly fatty foods showing up in healthier, low-fat versions recently. Evidently, someone has found a way to remove fat and replace it with purely theoretical particles, providing the minimum daily requirement for neutrinos.

Being a doctor, I try to eat food from healthy groups, like the "boneless, skinless" group and the "shreds of roughened wood" group. I have always considered Twinkies to be a leading example of food that is bad for you, namely the "high-calorie, heavy-cream-filled sponge cake" group.

This was before I learned about Low Fat Twinkies. "Low fat" in this case was a relative term. The new Twinkies, according to the Twinkie Hotline (the 800 number found on the wrapper), have 3 grams of fat in a package of two. (Nutritional scientists will tell you there is no such thing as a single Twinkie. Anyone who would eat one Twinkie is not going to carefully wrap up the other one for eating at a later date.) Fat-wise, this puts them in the same ballpark as three slices of bread or kernels of movie popcorn. While not technically a health food due to the cellophane packaging, they aren't bad.

As an observer of health trends, I felt it was my duty to conduct some research into the new Twinkies, especially if it meant I got to eat some. I used to eat Twinkies a lot, but I swore off them after being brainwashed into good nutrition during medical school. I have jealously eyed them in supermarkets and convenience stores ever since.

Now I had an excuse. Would these healthier Twinkies taste like the ones I remembered? Or would they taste like, well, like Twinkies with the Twink taken out?

Eager to find out, I put on my long white coat and went to the grocery store. I found the Twinkies on the Hostess rack, next to all the other snacks I remembered from my youth—cupcakes with squiggles on top, fruit pies shaped like burritos, and Sno-balls: small mounds of rubberized coconut that now come in designer pastel colors. Tears streaming down my face, I bought one twin-pack of Low Fat Twinkies and brought them home to my kitchen laboratory. I knew I had to be careful, particularly because of my recent problems with breakfast cereal. After years of eating cereal containing actual chunks of tree bark, I decided to bring home some Cap'n Crunch for my son. As many people know, Cap'n Crunch is a cereal consisting of tiny squares of sharpened fiberglass that are somehow impregnated with more sugar than if they were made entirely of sugar itself. Eating it is like eating tiny pieces of glazed sea coral. It was my favorite cereal as a kid, and it is wonderful.

My wife, however, thought it was a bad idea. I calmly pointed out that I ate Cap'n Crunch, and I still had a large number of my own teeth. I also reassured her that I was not an irresponsible parent, and that this was in fact 100 percent pure Cap'n Crunch, not the kind with the hideous "crunch berries" that stain the milk red.

Sadly, my son wasn't interested. He tried a few bites, played with the enclosed magic squirt pen, and then pushed it aside and asked for Cheerios. There was nothing I could do but finish that box myself, along with the 9 or 10 boxes I have purchased since, just in case he changes his mind.

Obviously, sweetened snack foods from my past were nothing to play around with. I was cautious as I tore open the package and took out a Twinkie. It looked just as I remembered, with the same pleasing weight and heft. The golden color was the same, with one darker, flattened side that still had the holes from the pneumatic cream-filling injector. It even left a thin coating of Twinkie skin stuck to the waxy cardboard, just as I remembered.

With the video camera running to document my research, I took a bite.

Medical research doesn't always bring bad news. My results show that Low Fat Twinkies taste surprisingly like the Twinkies I remember, essentially like damp Styrofoam packing material with a central core of sweetened library paste. They are wonderful.

I think my son might even like them, although I plan to stick to health food myself. I bet this box of 36 will last us for months.

I Just Play One on TV

I make a lot of fun of TV doctors. This is, of course, because I secretly want to be one. Even now, during a busy day of practice I will often drop what I'm doing and shout, "Get this man into emergency surgery right away!"

This can be alarming to someone who only came in for a sore throat. Still, I know it would be worth it if I could help just one person—one sick and needy person—get their picture on the ten o'clock news.

TV News Doctors

I hope that people aren't watching TV News Doctors to stay healthy. Watching News Doctors to stay healthy is like watching "Star Trek" to become a better astronaut, although in all fairness some episodes of "Star Trek" are pretty realistic compared to TV news.

TV is not the best place to get your medical care, and the reason is simple: For something to qualify as news on TV, you have to be able to take a picture of it. Usually this means showing a videotape of some object after the news has happened to it, like a burned-out building or a crashed airplane. This makes it hard for TV news to report on medical topics. No cameraman has ever been able to get a live on-the-scene action-cam shot of cholesterol.

Instead, some stations have hired TV News Doctors, who are mostly actual doctors who once took care of actual patients but don't any more. A few of them never really worked as doctors at all, staying in school just long enough to get the "M.D." behind their names. Calling these people "Doctor" is like calling Gerald Ford "President"—although technically correct, it is really more of a polite gesture.

Of course, if these News Doctors were actually going to report on medical problems they would have to show pictures of sick people, and this would mean one thing: poor ratings. Nobody wants to go to bed after seeing sick people on TV. Sometimes, just to get your attention, they might show a person in a wheelchair with an oxygen mask, which is the medical equivalent of a crashed airplane. Usually they just show people leaving buildings and having meetings, interspersed with shots of the TV News Doctor looking seriously concerned.

OPENING: Local news show begins, with loud, driving music full of electronic beeping sounds and heavy drum beats, while smiling pictures of caucasian news personalities are shown on the screen.

CUT TO:

Handsome Anchorman: Good evening. Tonight on "Live Eyewitness Action News Scene," we have exclusive pictures of a bunch of stuff after news has happened to it, along with some events we staged ourselves. But first, Dr. Marv Baleen, who is an actual doctor, has an important medical story that we all should be concerned about. Dr. Baleen?

News Doctor: Thank you, Brad. (Turns toward camera, concerned look on his face.) Tonight on "To Your Medical Health Line Watch and You:" Cryogenics, the story of people who freeze themselves. Seems crazy, but some people are doing just that. As you can see from these clips from old science fiction movies, there are people who are having themselves frozen in huge blocks of ice until later on, when they hope to thaw out. Fortunately, most of these people were already very sick. In fact, every one of them was dead and declined to be interviewed.

Still, for some of them, the cryogenic nightmare continues. In an exclusive report, we here at "To Your Medical Health Line Watch" have discovered that this process, freezing, is the very same one that caused thousands of injuries in this country during the '60s and '70s due to exploding pop bottles. Here are some pictures of people who have been hurt by exploding things. Because of serious injuries like this, most experts recommend avoiding freezing yourself. Here are a bunch of these experts leaving an important meeting. Ask your doctor if freezing is right for you. (Turns back toward anchorman.) Brad?

Handsome Anchorman: Dr. Baleen, that is a startling report. I haven't even seen a pop bottle for years.

News Doctor: Well, they're out there.

Handsome Anchorman: I have a spontaneous and unrehearsed question that I just happened to be wondering about. What about those plastic two-liter bottles? Do those also present a danger to our viewers?

News Doctor: I'm glad you asked that. (Turns toward camera, concerned look, etc., etc.) Here are exclusive pictures of some of those two-liter bottles lined up on grocery store shelves, and I have to say, Brad, it could happen. As this woman, now in a wheelchair and on oxygen, would probably agree.

Handsome Anchorman: Dr. Baleen, thank you for that alarming report, which has us all very concerned. We're lucky to have an actual doctor on our show to keep us informed about important health matters.

News Doctor: My pleasure. And, please, take care.

The scary thing about reports like these is that at least a few people take them seriously. Some of them really will ask their doctors, who will then look at them strangely. The patients will wonder why their doctors aren't keeping up with the latest medical literature, as shown on TV. Some of them will stop going to their doctors altogether, relying on TV News Doctors instead because, like everybody else, they want to be healthy.

But then I guess a lot of people want to be astronauts, too.

Doogie and The Moose

It's time to take a careful, objective look at doctor shows on TV. Why? So we can learn more about medicine and the way doctors work and live.

Just kidding. We will, however, learn a lot about TV.

There are two doctor shows now on TV: "Doogie Howser, M.D.," about a teenage genius who became a doctor at 16, and "Northern Exposure," about a doctor who must spend four years in Alaska to pay back an enormous medical school debt.

What can we learn by comparing these two shows?

In order to perform this intensive, complex analysis I went through a long and often difficult process.

Step 1

I went to medical school. I also went through internship and residency, although these are not technically required for this kind of program analysis.

Step 2

I watched 1 1/2 episodes of "Doogie Howser," concentrating exclusively on the program except for reading an occasional magazine and blocking out the sound during the really stupid parts.

Step 3

I watched at least as many episodes of "Northern Exposure." Well, I might have seen a few more of these. Maybe I watched each episode at least twice. I might even keep them on videotape, filed on my shelves next to the New England Journal of Medicine, but even if that were true I couldn't say so because it might possibly affect the objective nature of my research.

After a season of painstaking study, I have organized my data into clinical comparisons by subject, just like real scientists do. Here is what I learned:

Premise

"Northern Exposure" ("N.E.") is about a doctor who was forced to sign up for government-backed loans to finish school. Now, to honor his commitment, he must work in the wilds of Alaska instead of starting a lucrative private practice in New York. This kind of thing happens every year as the cost of medical education spirals upward.

"Doogie Howser, M.D." ("D.H.") is about a precocious teenager who finishes college while most of his classmates are still trying to remember the names of the different Ninja Turtles. It is unclear how he managed to rocket through medical school, which takes four years no matter how smart you are, but, hey, it could happen, at least on TV.

Main character

Joel Fleishman, the doctor in "N.E.," is a lovable mensch trying to make it in a foreign land, a place where moose roam the streets and the spring "ice break" is a major cultural event.

"D.H." is a know-it-all, smarty-pants wimpy kid just like the one you always wanted to beat the snot out of back in high school.

Supporting characters

"N.E.": The residents of Cicely, Alaska, are a group of eccentric, rugged individuals, with all of their quirks intact. Each has learned to survive in a climate that would send a lesser man, like Joel, packing. These people have learned to rely on each other, and they make us want to move to Alaska to be with them.

"D.H.": They all just love Doogie.

Romance

"D.H.": Doogie, as you might expect, has no problem getting babes, despite the fact that he looks like Howdy Doody only with more freckles.

During one episode Doogie was kissed by an internationally known fashion model, who was thanking him for helping her with a little eating-disorder problem.

I forget how many times this really happened to me during residency.

The bulimia episode was an attempt to present a socially relevant subject in a situation comedy. Of course, TV being what it is, it took Doogie about 30 minutes to solve the problem.

"N.E.": Somewhere during the first few episodes, Joel was dumped by his girlfriend back in New York. Small towns being what they are, it was roughly 30 minutes before this news was broadcast on the local radio station for everyone to hear.

Medical accuracy

"N.E.": Accurate. Joel deals with everyday problems like insomnia and vasectomy, and he handles his patients well. It is a glimpse into a true family practice, where not every problem has an answer. For serious things, backup is available from the specialists in Anchorage, although Joel can never convince any of the town folk to go there.

"D.H.": Accurate, but snotty and condescending. The doctors

randomly use medical jargon and then restate things in terms a nitwit could understand. In a serious problem, it is always Doogie who saves the day, all of the more experienced doctors presumably on vacation. I suspect the other interns routinely wish they could beat the snot out of him.

Spinoff potential

"N.E.": None. Well, maybe a nature show featuring the moose, but that's about it.

"D.H.": We can expect a number of related "properties." I imagine there will be a show for Doogie's slimy best friend Vinnie, a sex-crazed adolescent who, although he lives in a white, middle-class suburb, has a Brooklyn accent. I would also watch for a spinoff series featuring a group of bulimic fashion models.

Prognosis

"D.H.": A runaway hit, probably spawning a wave of "teenaged professional" shows for next season, like "Junior Logan, Attorney at Large," or "The Adventures of Sergeant Jimmy, L.A.P.D."

"N.E.": Dead. Two seasons as a midseason replacement may be all we see of this mature, intelligent show. In other words, it is just too good to make it on TV.

It almost makes me hope my research is wrong.

The TV Doctor Stethoscope Test

Another TV season, another new doctor show on TV. They show up each fall. I think there must be some sort of federal regulation that requires them to put a new doctor show on the air each year, no matter how bad it might be.

Most of these programs start out as midseason replacements, hoping to win a spot in the fall lineup. "Northern Exposure" started that way, and it became a big hit. Most of them fail horribly, disappearing from the schedule in a few short weeks.

One new show was "The Human Factor." I wanted to give an insightful, careful review of the show, but I had some trouble actually watching an entire episode. For one thing, it's an hour long. That means a significant commitment of time, a risky move considering the track record of doctor shows and the slim chance that it might not be terrible.

It also means that my attention tends to wander. A TV show has to be pretty good to keep me interested for 60 minutes. "Sesame Street" can usually do it; "The Human Factor," at least the first episode, didn't.

Most people think that, as a doctor, I would be in an excellent position to judge the quality of doctor shows on TV. They suppose I could use my knowledge of medicine and my experience working in clinics and hospitals to give a pretty accurate opinion of how realistic the show might be.

I guess that would work. Actually, I have always used a slightly different method for evaluating doctor shows: I judge them by the stethoscopes.

Because of this, my mind was already made up about "The Human Factor" when I saw the picture on the front of the "TV Week" magazine. There was the main character, a crusty, seasoned doctor with years of experience, a man who selflessly gave up his own practice to teach medical students, and he was wearing a stethoscope that looked like it came from a convenience store.

I have the picture on my bulletin board, mostly because it brings back memories of my own first stethoscope. My medical school gave one to each of us when we started our hospital work, and it was almost three days later when it fell apart, the metal chest piece dropping into the lap of my startled patient. It had a single, skinny tube like the one in the picture, which made it hard to listen through but easy to drape across the back of your neck, Hollywood-style. That's the way the doctor has it on in this picture, and to me, that says a lot about the show.

I know this seems like a dumb way to judge a TV program, but it can be remarkably accurate. Take "St. Elsewhere." When it first went on the air it was a great show. It showed hard-working young doctors dealing with common problems and difficult patients, and all of the characters had great stethoscopes. Later, when the ratings dropped, they made a few changes. The doctors started committing suicide and getting raped in prison, and the stethoscopes, among other things, suffered. By the time the plastic surgeon with AIDS was slashed by the vengeful, psychotic nurse, they had given up using any stethoscopes at all.

Judging from the picture, I have a bad feeling about "The Human Factor." I am afraid it will face the same problem that ruins most television shows. The quest for ratings will make it impossible to tell simple stories about everyday problems. Every condition will become a race against death. Eventually these shows become more like episodes of "Kojak" than doctor shows. That's why we won't see episodes about sore throats, or laryngitis, or insomnia, or even about someone dying comfortably at home.

"Northern Exposure," a big hit, covered all of those things, and that was just the first season. Of course, the doctor on that show always wears his stethoscope the right way, hanging down his chest like a tie. They even show him using it once in a while.

This ought to tell the networks something.

If shows like "The Human Factor" want to be big hits too,

they're going to have to focus on things people can relate to. Otherwise, they are just cop shows with white coats.

Oops—now I've spilled the beans.

Hollywood will know better now. Either they will start producing more shows that give an honest, realistic portrayal of doctors, or else they'll just hang better stethoscopes around their necks.

I guess we'll find out next fall.

Is Rex Morgan Alive or Dead?

I went on vacation a few weeks ago. I won't tell you where I went, but I will say this: It was far enough that they still had "Rex Morgan, M.D." on the comics page.

I wouldn't say that "Rex Morgan, M.D." was the main reason I wanted to become a doctor. In fact, I thought he was kind of a geek. I remember reading it when I was a kid. After it was dropped I figured the strip had ended, but there it was, still appearing in another paper in a different city.

Most of the things I remember about "Rex Morgan M.D." are still true. Like, for one thing, he hardly ever appeared in his own comic strip. All you ever saw was his name on the title. The actual day-to-day stories dealt with a bunch of loser characters that could never get their lives together. About every other week Dr. Morgan would step in, make a brief appearance and save them, solving their problems for them and allowing the story to move on to the next collection of losers.

That's exactly how it went during my vacation week. I never saw Rex until Sunday, the last day, when he made a cameo appearance and saved somebody from undergoing an unnecessary operation. You could almost understand it if these people were his patients—doctors are supposed to spend time helping them. But these characters in trouble, these people who could never even get dressed without asking him for advice—most of them were his friends! He liked them! Back then I remember thinking, "Geez, Rex, you're a cool guy, a doctor. You have it made! What are you doing hanging around with these dweebs?" This kind of life did nothing to reassure me that medicine was a great career.

When Rex finally did show up, he looked just like I remembered him—bland, square-shaped face, sharp chin, neatly-combed blue hair with a metallic sheen, and a dark brown suit colored just slightly outside the lines.

I recognized him right away, especially with the small, round mirror over his forehead. Rex Morgan always wore a head mirror, probably for the same reason that movie doctors wear them: so everybody can tell which one is the doctor. After all, the characters in "Rex Morgan" always looked pretty much alike. We are not dealing with great art here. You can tell the women apart because of their hairstyles, and you can usually tell the women from the men, but anything beyond that is a stretch.

Even though Rex was not a great influence on me, I still have one lasting effect from reading the strip: To this day, I cannot put on a head mirror without cracking up. Believe it or not, there are times when these things can be useful, only I don't dare put one on because it will suddenly occur to me that I must look exactly like Rex Morgan, M.D. I feel foolish.

Outside of mirrors, "Rex Morgan, M.D." had very little to do with medicine. This is despite the fact that it was created, as it turns out, by a real doctor. Dr. Nicholas P. Dallis, a psychiatrist, was the creator of several popular comic strips, including "Rex," "Apartment 3-G" and "Judge Parker." Dr. Dallis wrote the stories, but he evidently drew like a psychiatrist, forcing him to leave the art chores to somebody else.

As a psychiatrist, Dr. Dallis must have had plenty of material to work with. I wonder how his patients felt about his double career, especially knowing that their innermost secrets might possibly become the basis for a character in a comic strip. ("Look, Harold, this guy in the comics has the same little problem with feather dusters that you have!")

You can see why a psychiatrist would be envious. They spend years with guys like Harold, trying to work through their little quirks; Rex Morgan, M.D., could solve any problem in two weeks.

What a showoff. Well, let him keep his comic-page practice in some other city. Unless I go on vacation, I don't think I'll miss him a bit.

Doctor in Space, Action Figure on Earth

I wanted to be a doctor because I wanted to help people and because being a doctor looked cool on TV. There were a lot of great role models for doctors when I was growing up, like Dr. (Bones) McCoy on "Star Trek."

There is a new doctor in space. For the last seven years Gates McFadden has been playing Dr. Beverly Crusher on "Star Trek: The Next Generation," both on TV and in a new wave of Star Trek movies. The new show is a sequel to the original series, the most obvious differences being characters who wear actual uniforms instead of pajamas and who manage to maintain their weight from week to week.

I enjoy this show a lot, although I am not a "Trekkie," despite once having had my picture in a national magazine wearing pointy foam-rubber ears. When I learned that most of the cast was coming to town to do a play called "Every Good Boy Deserves Favour," I naturally had several questions, not the least of which was, "How can I talk to Gates McFadden?"

It turned out to be simple. The secret is not to call them yourself, but to have an editor from a major newspaper call for you. I can't stress this enough. If you call yourself, you will only end up talking to people who are paid to keep you away. My editor is not a "Trekkie" either, although he does keep a "Commander Data" action figure on his desk.

I wanted to tell McFadden that as a TV doctor, she's in a special position. Her character is an important role model for the doctors of tomorrow, even though the "Star Trek" line of action figures originally lacked a "Dr. Crusher."

As it turns out, I didn't have to tell her she's a role model. She knows. McFadden has given a lot of thought to her part as a doctor on a popular TV show, and, I am happy to report, she takes it very seriously.

"I hear from a lot of young people who say they want to go into medicine because of the show," she told me. "I also hear from doctors who enjoy the character of Dr. Crusher. A lot of them want my photo to put in their offices." I scratched "ask for photo" off my list and asked instead about her own views of the character.

"When I first started we talked a lot about what kind of doctor I would be. I loved the books of Oliver Sacks. I wanted to play that kind of character, a doctor who is open to different things and who has a sense of humor."

It always surprised me that she could portray a sensitive, caring doctor in the highly technical environment of TV space. "In the beginning, it was always the same thing. 'Quick, give him a hypo-spray.' The hypo-spray became like a panacea for everything that went wrong. I knew we needed to work on things like bedside manner.

"Now I always try to touch my patients physically, even if it's not in the script. Sometimes the writers will have me talking to someone else while working on a patient, and I always try to find another way. If I were the patient, I would find that annoying."

For someone who practices in the 24th century, McFadden thinks a lot about health-care issues of the 20th. "It's really a problem with our culture in general," she said. "More technology doesn't necessarily solve everything. We know now that the mind and spirit are just as important in healing."

I asked if playing a doctor on TV made people treat her differently. "Oh, I always try to demystify that quickly. I usually make a joke of it—'Well, I'm only a doctor in space. You'd need really good insurance before I could look at you.'

"Actually, it's most awkward when we have terminally ill children visiting the set. I feel so inadequate. They're looking at the tricorders and hypo-sprays, and I think, Oh, God, if only this wasn't pretend."

She is proud of the way "Star Trek" has addressed medical problems. "We have had episodes about cryonics, euthanasia and aging, although we still have a lot to cover. What about dentistry? What about people who are chronically ill? People are going to be living a lot longer, and we will have to help them deal with their pain."

Although the show is full of what she calls "technobabble," many of the principles and medical terms are real. We talked about genetic drift, neurobiology, and current medical research.

"What I would love is to do a story like *Awakenings* where we can reach people who have an unknown disease and revive them, giving them a new level of consciousness."

The future seems to be in good hands. I wouldn't push my son into medicine, but I'm glad he can have the kind of role model that I did.

And I am happy to report an official "Dr. Crusher" action figure is now available in toy stores everywhere.

"You should write about that," she told me. "I always thought it was discrimination, because they had dolls of all the men. After all, if we're going to be examples for our kids, we might as well include a doctor."

After talking to McFadden, I plan to buy one. I might even lend it to my son.

I Was a TV News Doctor

Here's something I want to get out in the open, just in case I am ever nominated for attorney general: I was a TV News Doctor.

Not just once, either. I have been on local news stations twice—all right, three times, on two stations. I'm not proud of this. I'm only now reaching the point where I can talk about it without making excuses or blaming Clark DePaolis, my evil twin.

Years ago I auditioned with a talent agency for a television job. I was quickly eliminated. I wanted to talk about having checkups and quitting smoking; they wanted stories about deadly medical blunders and household objects that could secretly kill you.

Later, when TV reporters asked me to appear in medical stories, I agreed. I thought I could give people some important medical information. Plus, like most people, I really wanted to know what I looked like on TV.

The first time was a report on diet pills. It focused on two new medicines for weight loss, which were basically just the same old amphetamines with new, flashier names. I went on TV and said they were dangerous and habit-forming, and that patients should concentrate on exercise instead. This was followed by footage of trim bodies working out, while the anchorperson said, "Diet pills—new hope for people who just can't lose weight." This is 90 percent of the population, the exact number of people who called their doctors the next morning to ask for some.

The next time was for a story on addiction. The reporter asked me to talk about caffeine withdrawal. I figured they wanted me to tell their viewers how to cut down and stay healthy. Later I learned that the story was really about some woman who drinks many gallons of soda pop every day. They wanted to show her drinking pop while someone with an advanced medical degree said what anyone would

87

say: "Boy, that's a lot of pop." This startling report also featured other cases of trivial, made-up addictions, like a psychologist who said she was addicted to red licorice and a man who was so incredibly addicted to books that he actually bought more without reading them(!).

The last time I was on TV was for a story about vitamins. Through extensive research of an old copy of Time magazine, this reporter had learned that certain vitamins might help prevent heart disease. The report was already written, and all they wanted was someone in a white coat to repeat the main sound bite: "Vitamins prevent heart attacks."

I knew the vitamin story was hype, and this is what I said for the tape: "Some research does suggest that certain vitamins may help prevent heart disease, BUT no one knows if this is really true, and taking megadoses of any vitamin is not a good idea." You will never in a million years guess where they edited that sentence, abruptly cutting off the audio and leaving me flapping my lips on the screen like a mime doing bass impressions. Even I—a person whose knowledge of TV journalism was gained mostly from the movie "Broadcast News," where TV reporter William Hurt fakes tears for the camera—even I knew this was a hatchet job.

Now I know how I look on TV—I look shorter and kind of stupid.

Obviously, most people don't watch TV News Doctors for medical advice, but for the entertainment value of seeing a doctor act like a goof. There's nothing wrong with that—I'm sure that's why people bought this book—but it's important to know they aren't going to get any real advice on staying healthy. Even stations with excellent reporters have medical news that is just one step away from reports on Loni Anderson's latest anxiety medicine or fancy computer graphics showing John Wayne Bobbitt's reattachment surgery.

Some local stations are now declaring their 5 p.m. shows to be "Family News," without sensational stories that are only meant to shock and titillate viewers.

If stations really did this, people might finally get some medical news that matters, and I wouldn't have to be afraid to tell people that I was a TV News Doctor. Maybe I'll even go on TV News again someday—probably right after I'm nominated for attorney general.

Bad Medicine

Everyone knows that some things doctors do can later turn out to be big mistakes. The medical treatments from hundreds of years ago are now routinely mocked, like the operation where they shave off half of your hair and drill holes in your skull to let out the bad demons. This had not been done for years until it was done to Ronald Reagan.

A lot of our current medical practices will also seem ridiculous years from now. Actually, some of them are pretty silly even today. For example, when Hippocrates said, "First, do no harm," he could never in his wildest dreams have imagined anything like liposuction.

New Forms of Birth Control

Most people think they know everything about birth control. A lot of them are now parents. There have been startling breakthroughs in the contraception field recently. This is an exciting topic, even without illustrations, so let's get right to it.

Condoms

In the last few years condoms have gained widespread respectability. This means that they have now been mentioned on every television sitcom, usually by obnoxious child actors. Condoms have become much easier to get, although they are no easier to get on. They now hang on a rack at Target, right next to the Q-tips, allowing people to buy them without having to say the word "prophylactic" to some nosy pharmacist.

Most condom advertising is aimed at women. New colors, designer labels and fashion prints are now available. There are even "bikini" condoms—women's fashion underwear in tasteful designer colors, with a built-in condom already in place. These products allow women to feel more comfortable with condoms, while creating a new market for celebrity endorsements in TV commercials, which most stations will refuse to show.

Female condoms

Most new birth control is a result of the shifting balance of the sexes in medicine. More women are becoming doctors, letting them guide research and development of new methods.

This also makes them less likely to accept some of the older methods designed by men, like the IUD, a device that for years was hydraulically loaded into women's bodies, producing the same effect in the uterus as a road construction crew on an interstate highway.

The most sensational new development has been the female condom. (This will probably be followed by the Women's Football League and movies featuring The Three Stoogettes.) Scientists invented the female condom in an effort to create a birth control device that looks even more ridiculous than regular old condoms. Picture a regular condom, or actually a box of 24. Then imagine the plastic bag it came wrapped in, and there you have it. For most women, the major problem is finding a wallet big enough to keep it in.

These new products give women the same control over conception that they have traditionally enjoyed over sex. After all, the most effective birth control occurs at the front door. ("Thanks. I had a nice time. No, don't call. I'll call you.")

Oral contraceptives

The pill has now been around for 30 years, but not much has changed. Most advancements have been in the area of package shapes. As most people know, the pill does not come in little bottles like other pills. Now, in addition to the standard ovals and rectangles, there are packages in the shape of rhomboidal tetrahedrons, along with the new "M.C. Escher" package design that never seems to run out.

The other big change is in the strength of the medicine. Ever since the first pills, which contained enough estrogen to cause menstruation in inanimate objects, doctors have been lowering the dose. Now, besides the mini-pills and the micro-mini-pills, there is the infinitesimal-pill, containing the smallest dose of estrogen that can still be detected by the naked eye.

"Roseanne"

Although not technically a birth control device, watching one episode has been shown to lead to a dramatic drop in sexual drive, good for about three days of abstinence in most men. Women may achieve the same effect from watching "Geraldo."

91

RU-486

This is the famous "French abortion pill," which causes quick and safe termination of pregnancy. There are few side effects, other than a sudden appreciation for Jerry Lewis movies. RU-486 has been at the center of a tremendous legal battle waged by male lawyers and judges. Manufacturer's research shows that the drug is safe and should be sold in this country, but company executives point out that continuous market-share surveys have shown industrywide trend analysis blah blah blah. Basically, nobody wants to wake up and find 500,000 individual postcards from "right to life" groups on their doorstep.

Norplant

This is a set of six medicated rods that are implanted in a woman's arm. They provide safe and effective birth control, as long as someone has sex with that arm.

Birth control for men

Now that women have a say, there are several new methods being developed for use on men. Most of them involve doing something to the male genitalia. This is not as easy as it sounds. While females only release an ovum every 28 days, males are producing sperm constantly, sometimes to the exclusion of everything else.

Ultrasound treatments, painful sperm cord injections, and female hormones have all been tried on selected male subjects, typically medical students. Results have been discouraging, but researchers seem determined to press on, hoping to find just the right combination of discomfort and inconvenience that will give men the same options that women have had. After all these years, it is only fair.

The Power Tool Approach to Weight Loss

Ever since I started medical school I have been keeping a handy reference list of things I don't want done to me.

Liposuction quickly made the list, even though I have never actually seen it performed. For me, liposuction has always been one of those things, like a root canal, that I am willing to pass up on faith, with very few details.

Still, you can imagine how thrilled I was to find a videotape in the mail called "Liposuction Surgery." It contains actual footage of the procedure, and I can safely say it is one of the most disgusting things I have ever seen.

I used to think liposuction was just a silly, harmless diversion for pudgy rich people, but that was before I had seen the tape. It was sent to me by a dermatologist friend of mine who shows it to patients interested in liposuction. So far, he hasn't had any takers, which tells you something about this tape.

It starts with a talk by a plastic surgeon, who explains that patients must have realistic expectations. "We can smooth out the lumps," she warns, "but we can't make you a model." Of course, most of these same patients were attracted by plastic surgery ads featuring photos of women who have the same total body-fat content as one Oreo cookie.

Next an actual patient stands naked while the doctor, showing great sensitivity and concern, draws all over the woman's thighs with a Magic Marker. She marks a series of lines, circles and "X's" to "mark specific areas of fat concentration"—areas the patient could have easily pointed out if she'd been asked.

The patient, who now looks like a large weather map, is then placed on a table and covered with green sheets, just like in real surgery. Anesthesia is given, and the surgeon makes a small incision over the "problem areas." Then a sharp metal tube like a curtain rod is inserted under the skin, and "the powerful suction machine is turned on."

What follows next can only be described as lipo-massacre. I'll keep this on a certain level for those of you eating breakfast, but I can tell you that there are characters wearing hockey masks in low-budget teen-exploitation movies who show more care with sharp instruments.

Suffice it to say that the tube is moved back and forth in "a piston-like motion" to suck up the fat. I was always taught to be careful with power tools, but the doctor in this tape uses her Craftsman 2000 XT model variable-speed liposuctor with auto reverse as if she had never been to shop class.

Meanwhile, the patient's skin, which has evidently grown accustomed to these fat deposits, is putting up a valiant fight to keep them. This requires several burly assistants to keep the patient on the table while the surgeon works.

Actually, "surgeon" is not really a good title for a person in this job, which is basically the same thing the plumber does when the drainpipe gets clogged. The term "suction," on the other hand, turns out to be pretty accurate for a procedure that sounds like a bunch of grade-school boys playing with gelatin.

In the next hideous scene, as the narrator puts it, "fat can be seen moving through the transparent tube." This must be a popular spot to stop viewing. Most people would rather see something less graphic, like the films of gruesome car accidents they show in driver's ed.

"No more than 2,000 cc's are removed at any one time," the doctor says finally, showing us what looks like an extremely heavy two-liter soda bottle. The fat is taken somewhere and discarded. No one will tell me where.

The tube is removed, the incision is sewn shut and several miles of gauze is wrapped around the patient. This is to hide the fact that her thighs now look like gallons of ice cream with one scoop taken out. Recovering takes about four weeks, slightly longer than it takes to re-cover a love seat.

After seeing this tape, "liposuction" has moved to the top of my "don't do" list, underlined and with several added stars. I can't imagine who would have this done to them on purpose if there was a way out, especially since they could accomplish the same thing by eating less and taking a brisk walk every day. In a time when so many people go without even basic health care, it is sad to see valuable medical resources wasted on troublesome fatty deposits.

Unfortunately, more people will be going under the curtain rod soon. The implant business has suffered a few setbacks, and some plastic surgeons are going back to featuring liposuction in their advertising instead ("Buy the friendly thighs").

I can only assume that these people haven't seen this tape. Either that, or they really enjoy root canals.

Nicotine Gets under Your Skin

There are a lot of questions about nicotine patches, thanks mainly to countless TV and magazine ads that urge "ask your doctor." Let's take a look at some of those questions, along with—as a special bonus—the answers.

Q: What's the deal with these patches, anyway?

A: Medicine patches are nothing new. They have been used for blood pressure and hormones for years, usually by people who forget to take their pills. These people go along with the patches, mostly because they don't really believe they work. No one really believes that they can soak up medicine through their skin like a paper towel, no matter what their doctor says.

Q: Do they work?

A: Nicotine patches are 100 percent absolutely guaranteed to perform their main function, getting nicotine into your body.

Q: But isn't nicotine bad for you?

A: No worse than any carcinogenic amphetamine.

Q: Then how can they help people quit smoking?

A: Patches provide another way to get the nicotine, just like nicotine gum did. People can then go without cigarettes, allowing them to still be addicted without having yellow teeth and smelling like a carpet in a bowling alley. The main advantage of the patch over gum is that you can fall asleep without getting it stuck in your hair.

Q: How long can you use them?

A: Through careful research, the manufacturers have determined that these patches are safe for a period of time up to, but not longer than, patients are willing to pay for them. Doctors disagree. They know that sooner or later everyone has to give up the patches. Many people get through this difficult time by substituting other sources of nicotine, like cigarettes.

Q: Are there any side effects?

A: The main side effect seems to be having your body covered with large red spots, making it look like you have been attacked by a love-starved octopus. These are permanent only some of the time.

Q: Are they expensive?

A: By an incredible coincidence, one patch a day costs exactly the same as smoking one and a half packs a day. (This is without the added cost of chemotherapy, which comes later.) This seems like a lot until you compare it to other ways of harming yourself, like motorcycles or hang gliders. Of course, these other activities are nowhere near as efficient as smoking. A lot of people survive hang-gliding.

Q: Does insurance pay for patches?

A: Usually not, which upsets a lot of smokers until they realize that they are already getting a significant price break on their health insurance, especially since they are the ones who will be using up most of the money for respirators and oxygen tanks later.

Q: Can someone still smoke while wearing the patch?

A: They most certainly may, although they might have an immediate heart attack and die. Although nothing breaks the smoking habit like a few nights in intensive care, manufacturers recommend against it.

Q: Are the patches for everyone?

A: The drug companies say no, advising doctors to carefully select only patients who have skin covering some portion of their body. While not for everyone, they may be the answer for people who have tried several times to quit and are fed up with smoking. Not every smoker is happy being a helpless tool of large tobacco conglomerates, who make millions off their noxious products. Patches were developed for those people who prefer to be helpless tools of large pharmaceutical companies instead.

Q: Is it necessary to visit a doctor?

A: Yes, it is essential to have a complete history and thorough examination by a physician, who will then write a prescription anyway. Doctors know that nicotine patches are bad for you, but are still safer than actually smoking. Besides, this system keeps dangerous substances like nicotine under tight control. After all, it's not like any 16-year-old can just walk in and buy nicotine at the corner convenience store.

Q: What about hypnosis?

A: To be successful, the subject must be extremely weak-willed and suggestible. In fact, in this pamphlet I am reading right now, it says that most people . . . most people . . . getting a little . . . sleepy . . . tick . . . tock . . . WHY, YES, HYPNOSIS IS AN EXCELLENT WAY TO QUIT SMOKING. HYPNOSIS CAN WORK WONDERS. ASK YOUR DOCTOR.

Arm Hair on Your Head

People are always asking me, "How come you never write about the health care crisis that has seriously burdened our economy and threatens to overwhelm the entire system of medical care in this country?" They also ask, "What can I do about hair loss?"

What I tell them is to watch more late-night TV. That's where a lot of the really important baldness research is going on. Almost every night these results are gathered into informative 30-minute programs designed for the concerned and thinning consumer.

I know this because I fell asleep on the couch one night during the "Tonight Show" (not a comment on Jay Leno's performance). When I awoke I discovered I had left network TV, where commercials are conveniently spaced apart by 2 or 3 minutes of actual program, and was now watching "Info-mercial TV," where the programs and commercials have mutated and somehow combined, probably through cold fusion.

What I saw was a bunch of active men doing a variety of vigorous, active things like swimming and mountain climbing. At first I thought they must all be related—it was like stumbling onto some weird video family reunion. Then I realized that the reason they all looked alike was that they all wore large, furry rodents on their heads.

This was "The Hair Club," a late-night program where bald men could turn for help. These men were obviously very happy to be in the club. They kept telling each other how sad they had been before, when they were bald, and how great life was now that they had hairy objects attached to their heads. One of them was extremely happy—not only was he the president of the club, but he was also a member, as demonstrated by the fact that he had the largest rodent.

So now, when people ask, I tell them to wait until everyone else is asleep and tune in "The Hair Club."

Of course, not everyone is satisfied with a rodent. Some people want more. They want real hair, not just a pelt. These are the people who then ask me about "the medicine."

Actually, no one really ever comes right out and asks. Instead, they try to casually work it into the conversation, often while making fun of somebody else. "Look at that guy," they say, pointing at a passing scalp-impaired person. "Nice melon. Ha ha. Maybe he should make an appointment to get some of 'the medicine.' Ha ha. Say, that stuff doesn't really work, does it?"

What they are asking about is Minoxidil, the only FDA-approved medical treatment for baldness. Not that anyone can just say the name out loud. The TV commercials make it seem like it requires national security clearance to get a prescription.

"Ask your doctor," is all they say, nodding knowingly at the camera.

"Hey, this must be some powerful stuff," people are supposed to think, "because they can't even say the name on TV."

And it's not just men, either: There are now Minoxidil ads with women in them, who nod knowingly at the camera. These new ads are so vague they could be for feminine hygiene products.

Let me try to answer "the question:" Does it work? The answer is: yes, kind of. It works as well as many other personal grooming products, like the ones that promise to make your teeth "whiter than white" or make your private parts smell "as fresh as a summer's eve."

Take a look at your arm. See the little, fine hairs growing there? You may have to turn it a bit, trying to catch the light in a certain way. There, see the faint, tiny hairs growing there? Those are the kind of hairs that Minoxidil can give you. They will stay as long as you keep using the medicine, at about $55 a month. When you stop, they fall out.

Does anybody really want arm hair growing on their head? Evidently, the answer is yes. No matter how silly, a lot of people believe it would still look better than baldness. Some people are will ing to spend any amount of money for a chance to have hair, any hair, where there is now wide open scalp.

Which is probably OK, because insurance companies don't pay for hair-loss treatments, and this will pump thousands of private dollars into the health care industry, helping to ease the crisis that threatens to overwhelm the entire system of medical care in this country.

There. Now people won't have to ask.

Like Sheep to the Pharmacy

I like taking my dog to the vet. I certainly enjoy it a lot more than she does. I can tell because as soon we pull into the parking lot she throws all four of her legs into rigid extensor-lock position, her paws leaving skid marks as I drag her through the door.

Once inside the little room, my vet and I always spend time comparing our jobs. We treat some of the same diseases. I recognize most of the medications in the cabinet. The equipment is not that different from the stuff at my office, except for the elbow-length rubber gloves and this large metal clamp-type thing that I don't even want to know what it's for. In fact, except for the stainless steel tables, I feel right at home.

That's one reason why I was surprised by a recent story about the new cancer-fighting drug, Levamisole. In a dramatic medical breakthrough, the medicine was found to reduce the chances for recurrence of colon cancer in certain people. Although it is expensive, about $1,495 for a year's supply, the drug can be a life-saver.

My vet was surprised, too. He knows all about Levamisole. Vets have been prescribing the drug for 20 years to kill intestinal worms in sheep, although when he prescribes the drug it costs only $14.95 a year, one one-hundredth the cost for humans.

This price difference came to light when an Illinois woman who was being treated for cancer happened to take a look at the bottle while giving worm pills to her sheep. I'm sure she was surprised, too, especially after paying her pharmacy bill.

At first this seems to make sense. After all, sheep don't have a lot of money. They don't really care that they have worms. Veterinary medicines are generally a bit cheaper than their human counterparts, even if the only difference is in the packaging. Sometimes the actual pills are bigger ("horse pills," i.e., the size of a small horse), but usually the medicine is the same as the human stuff, made by the same company in the same factory.

That means that this incredible price boost for Levamisole can only be based on what people are willing to pay.

Colon cancer is the second-leading cause of cancer deaths in this country. Most of these patients already have been through some frightening experiences—surgery, radiation treatments, chemotherapy—and they are willing to pay anything for a chance to prevent their cancer from returning. It is hardly fair to take advantage of them this way.

Unfortunately, drug pricing has little to do with fairness. Norplant, an implantable, five-year birth-control medicine, costs about $5 in Finland. In this country, where people are willing to pay about $10 a month for birth control pills, or $600 over five years, Norplant, by an incredible twist of marketing fate, costs about $600. Nicotine patches, by another bizarre coincidence, cost almost exactly the same as smoking one and a half packs of cigarettes a day, the level where the addiction is hardest to break on your own.

In this kind of supply and demand, prices are based on need. No one would pay anything for a 10-pound chunk of Levamisole, unless of course they had colon cancer. Then they are held for ransom.

Not everyone can afford to pay. Some people are taking their prescriptions to their veterinarian, asking them to supply the medicine at a more reasonable price. It would actually be cheaper to buy a couple of sheep and hope they get worms, just so you could share their medicine. And that's not even counting the extra income the wool would bring.

Johnson & Johnson, the manufacturer, claims that it needs the money to cover its extensive research costs. It says this even though the most important research was done by the National Cancer Institute, which is funded by tax dollars from you and me and the patients who now need the drug to keep their cancer from returning. Besides, the company has been selling this stuff at a profit for 25 years. There should be enough money to buy each one of their lab oratory geeks two clipboards instead of one, and still have plenty of cash left for ice cream afterward.

What this kind of money really buys is the new ad campaign—the new marketing, new package, the snappy name and the millions of little trinkets for cancer doctors across the country.

Doctors are unlikely to accept them. Cancer experts, not normally a feisty bunch, have been up in arms about Levamisole. One of them, Dr. Charles Moertel from the Mayo Clinic in Rochester, Minnesota, was indignant at one national meeting, calling the price difference "unconscionable." Moertel, part of the team that helped the drug win FDA approval, said that the company promised to market it at a "reasonable" cost, a promise that quickly became just so much mutton.

Of course, even sheep may not have it so good for long. Some health insurance companies have started offering policies for pets. So far most of these policies have gone to annoying little yapping poodles with ribbons on their ears, but someday the benefits may be extended to farm animals. If that happens, you can bet that cheap Levamisole will be a thing of the past.

Fat-Zapping Lasers

Recently, a plastic surgeon at a local hospital used a laser to remove some fat from the waist of a male patient. This was the first operation to combine the cutting edge of laser technology with the American mania for fat reduction.

According to a news release, about two pounds of fat were removed in the 45-minute operation. By local hospital rates, this surgery must have cost at least $700, or approximately $350 a pound.

It seems like a lot of money to pay, but people have been shelling out this kind of money for years on health spas, diet plans, nutritional supplements and the kind of exercise equipment advertised on late-night TV. At least with surgery there are definite, tangible results. When the operation is over, if you don't mind the mess, you could hold those two pounds of fat in your hands. That's something the "gut-buster" could never give you.

On the other hand, except for the times a "gut-buster" threw a spring or slammed a door on somebody, most of these "get-thin-quick" plans are harmless. The most bizarre diet plans, like the eat-30-grapefruit-a-day diet, are impossible to follow for any length of time, and most of the protein supplements taste so bad that hardly anybody can finish a can of them. The only thing lost is money, or in the sadder cases, lots of money.

The risks of laser-liposuction, however, are the same as for any surgery. General anesthesia, while statistically quite safe, carries a certain risk. The laser technology makes the fat-pulling process a little neater, but does nothing to lessen these risks. Somehow, I am not reassured by the phrase "only a little blood loss."

But you have to consider the area in question: According to the story, the fat was taken from the "love handles" on both sides of the patient's waist, an area that has traditionally plagued men who wish to appear younger than their years. Men have no "love" for these small lumps of fat that hang just above the belt line, and some of them would do just about anything to get rid of them.

Anything within reason, of course. Without some kind of surgical procedure it would be necessary to burn up about 7,000 calories to get rid of those same two pounds. This would mean taking a 2-mile walk every day for almost a whole month. You can't expect busy people to put out that kind of effort just to lose a couple of pounds, especially when there is a new surgical procedure that can do the same thing, with no effort other than writing out a check.

By the look of things, this new operation will become a big seller in plastic surgery offices around the country. It's fast, getting patients in and out of the hospital in under a day. It might be a little embarrassing to be a liposuction patient, but hospital records are confidential. The procedure is expensive, but the basic premise of plastic surgery is that money never has to stand in the way of beauty, even lots and lots of money.

If the doctor who performed this operation is right, laser-lipo will spread throughout the more affluent areas of the country. People will shed their embarrassment and start comparing their tiny laser-beam scars at cocktail parties and country clubs everywhere. "Love handles" will go the way of love letters, and men and women who never walk any farther than the refrigerator will have slim waistlines.

More patients will be leaving hospitals a few pounds lighter, a lot poorer, but really no better than they were before.

Dog Surgery

Both my dog and I were happy to learn about a recent decision to cut back on using animals in medical school classes.

Although I went to dog surgery a few times as a student, I can't remember learning anything except the fact that most dogs, like most people, don't want surgery. This was obvious by the way the instructors had to hold them down during the anesthesia.

If it had been up to us, we would have let them go. The survival rate for medical student surgery is very low—zero, in fact. Most medical students will never become surgeons; in our hands, even putting in an IV was a risky adventure. For us, going to dog surgery was like taking notes while watching Benji being run over by a lawn mower.

I thought about this last summer, when my own dog needed surgery. She tore a cruciate ligament in her knee, the same sports-related injury that happens to many NFL running backs when they are on the practice field and suddenly see a squirrel. She bolted off at about Mach 6, darting over a grassy knoll and out of sight. According to the vet, she probably stepped in a hole, although with my dog it's possible the squirrel overpowered her. Either way, she came back on only three legs, the fourth dangling beneath her like warm spaghetti.

I watched her operation, being careful not to handle any sharp objects myself given my record (0-2) in dog surgery. Things are generally more relaxed in veterinary operations. For example, while the surgeon wears sterile gloves, scrubs and a mask, other people in the room can be in their normal clothes. This meant for once I would not be kicked out of an operation for touching my nose.

Although I have seen a lot of surgery, I have never watched an operation on a loved one. I don't recommend it. You start to question

107

every little thing, worrying when the surgeon grunts or when that the flap on the oxygen tank stops moving up and down.

Orthopedic surgery is not a delicate business. In fact, many orthopedic surgical instruments are in reality shop-grade power tools. Watching some orthopedic procedures is like watching a longshoreman boning a chicken. I still remember the sound it made when my dog's knee was pried open to reveal the tattered ligament inside, although my wife has asked me not to re-create it when I tell this story at dinner.

Still, the surgery went well, and afterward her veterinarian was careful to give me some rules for her recovery. Any human who has had knee surgery knows that a careful, step-by-step rehabilitation program is important in regaining strength and getting back to normal, and the same is true for dogs:

Week 1

Patient lies on her side like dead raccoon on the highway, whimpering at movement of air currents around injured leg. Idiot owner, who thinks he knows better because he has medical degree, removes some of bandage to make leg more comfortable. Owner then calls vet when part of leg without bandage swells to size of Dodge Grand Caravan.

Week 2

Final bandages removed. Leg appears to be raw turkey drumstick left in the sun for two weeks, only with worse smell. Owner tries to inspect wound, worried that stitches are opening. Owner accidentally opens stitches.

Weeks 3-6

Patient is confined to house, hobbling around on three legs and breaking several world records for indoor track events. Learns to hold up injured leg in pathetic attempt to beg for snacks.

Week 7

Start Active Rehabilitation, Phase 1. Patient takes first careful steps outside, carefully touching paw to ground while testing strength and stability until owner relaxes grip on leash. Phase 2: Spots another squirrel in the next yard. Charges off at near-sonic speed while barking loudly, ignoring frantic screams from owner. Stops to pee in neighbor's yard.

We never learned about recovery in dog surgery during medical school, mostly because none of our patients recovered.

Luckily, despite my help, my dog has. She was back on her knee in about the same time it takes a lizard to grow an entire new leg, something I will definitely keep in mind the next time I choose a household pet. She has even been able to return to strenuous activities like barking at passing airplanes and sleeping on piles of clothing.

As for me, I have seen enough dog surgery. I'm glad the university is putting a stop to it, saving on both money and dogs.

Besides, there are other ways to teach medical students. We used to practice on each other for interviewing and blood-drawing skills. Doing the same thing for surgery class would help future doctors remember that most people, and dogs, would rather not have surgery at all.

Medicial Impressions

These days people don't like doctors in general, although they might like their own doctor well enough. On the whole, doctors have a reputation for being pompous, arrogant, and condescending, even when they don't have special "MD" license plates.

While not as popular as they once were, people still like doctors better than lawyers, who are universally despised. Even a doctor who writes columns about space alien abductions and cartoon characters could theoretically help you if he happened to find you on the side of the road after an accident, whereas most lawyers would just sue you for obstructing traffic and wrongful bleeding.

Was Your Doctor a Major Geek?

Whenever I convince someone that I actually went to medical school, they always want to know one thing: Was their own doctor ever a major total geek?

The answer, tragically, is yes.

There is no better way to describe your average medical student. Who but a geek would bring a pathology textbook to their parents' anniversary party? Or study microbiology slides during intermission at a Broadway musical? Who else would recite the names of bio-chemical enzymes while waiting for their date to come out of the bathroom? Remember, these are people who took out federal loans so they could afford to have hospital interns ordering them to do demeaning, even disgusting things.

Even if a person were not a major geek when they got there, medical school would soon turn them into one. I started medical school with several people who seemed pretty cool, at least to me, but after a few short months they were well on their way to becoming complete dweebs. Some went willingly, some were dragged kicking and screaming, but all of them ended up in the same general place—geek city.

I thought about this at my 10-year reunion from medical school last year. I was sitting in a room full of neurologists, surgeons and anesthesiologists, but I wasn't seeing them that way. I saw the guy who got into trouble for breaking into the science library—not to steal anything, but so that he could squeeze in a few more hours of studying after closing time. Across from him was the man who once crawled across an office floor on his hands and knees to beg for a passing grade in one class. (He seemed very sincere from my vantage point, crawling along there beside him.) There was the woman who spent most of her medical student career making huge, elaborate charts in four colors of ink, and several others who used to bring themselves nearly to physical blows fighting over the chairs in the first row of the auditorium.

They are doctors now, respected members of their communities. Back then, believe me, they were geeks. We all were.

I know most people would like to think that their doctor was always the competent, sensitive provider they see in the office now. They want to believe their doctor spoke Latin as a child, and interpreted MRI scans at the fifth-grade science fair.

The truth is that no one is born knowing this stuff. At one time your doctor, whoever he or she may be, knew exactly as much about medicine as you do right now. Actually, they once knew even less, probably because they were concentrating on getting their underpants on with the picture of Mickey Mouse in the front.

This realization can be frightening, particularly as you get older and sicker, but it shouldn't be. Everyone starts out at the same place, knowing nothing about anything. Someone else has to teach them, and that's why we have institutions for higher learning like medical school and the College of Comic Book Knowledge.

So please, the next time you see a bunch of doctors on some street corner, try not to tease them. Remember, becoming major total geeks was just their way of coping.

Besides, no one says they have to stay geeks forever. There were people at the reunion who finished medical school and went on to live full, rewarding lives, maybe even taking up a hobby or going to movies. Some of them even left their pathology books at home, or at least in the trunk.

As for me, I was busy trying to remember the names of classmates while reliving some of the great old times we used to have in medical school, like groveling. Good thing I made sure to wear old pants.

113

L.A. Medicine

It's time to take a look at some exciting new trends in health care, as conveniently displayed on outdoor billboards. Normally, to cover this topic you would have to 1) make a thorough, careful review of current medical literature, with special emphasis on recent trends in molecular and biologic theory, or, if you are lazy, 2) go to California.

I recently got back from Los Angeles, City of the Drive-By Shootings, and I can tell you that life on the West Coast is undergoing a major social upheaval. For one thing, sandwiches no longer come with alfalfa sprouts, having been narrowly edged out in a statewide referendum by tiny pieces of shaved carrot.

Bold advances are also taking place in the field of outdoor medical advertising. California doctors use billboards to advertise their practices and get new patient referrals. Here in the Midwest you rarely see billboards for medical care, except for signs with huge close-up photos of chiropractors, making them look like balloons in the Macy's parade.

In California, however, it is not unusual to be driving along and suddenly find yourself facing some other enormous body part. For example, billboards for "The Endoscopic Institute, the center for minimally invasive surgery," are covered with the smooth, taut abdomen of a top fashion model, with one tiny Band-aid near her belly button. None of my own internal organs could have been removed through such a small opening, but fashion models are not the same as actual people.

In Los Angeles they have billboards for every kind of medical specialty, even some that don't really exist. They offer health care from pain management to hair transplants, which are also quite painful. In fact, there seems to be a lot of interest in pain, which is odd for a place with so many swimming pools and expensive foreign cars. Maybe it's because of all the tattoo parlors.

They even have ads for a team of crack pain management doctors and nurses called "the Painkillers." On the sign they are wearing jumpsuits and carrying large pieces of high-tech anti-pain equipment, like Ghostbusters in white. Their number is "1-800-800-PAIN." I wanted to call, but I happened to be driving a rental car, the only cars in California without cellular phones.

As we know from TV, the lawyers on "L.A. Law" deal with real-life subjects like sex, divorce and sex with divorce lawyers. L.A. Medicine, on the other hand, deals mainly with goofy ideas for ridiculous medical treatments. Why else would they have signs for "Aura Soma, the Science of Color Therapeutics"? People in Los Angeles visit the Nutritional Therapist like the rest of us go to the dentist. They stop by the medical doctor on the way home from the Aroma Therapist, just before their appointment for Hair Protein Analysis. Some billboards even offer one-stop medical shopping for busy patients, like the ads for one progressive clinic that offers the four most important health care specialties in California: "All the pieces of the total health care picture: internal medicine, chiropractic, acupuncture and HIV care."

All of this would be a lot less scary if California wasn't the home of every major social trend in the last 100 years, from skateboards to hideous "retro" fashions like bell bottoms. For some reason, California always gets to decide what the rest of the country will be doing next year. This is frightening. Remember, these are people who elected Ronald Reagan as their leader four times. This is a city where the major newspaper, the *Los Angeles Times,* runs ads on the sports page for "a leading specialist" who offers surgery to enlarge certain parts of the male anatomy. ("Dreams do come true. Men only.")

I think the problems come from living in a place with so much money and so much poverty at the same time. Life everywhere in America is unfair, but nowhere is this so obvious as in Los Angeles. L.A. drivers have to be careful not to park their Porsches on top of homeless people living in their parking spaces. You can live like this for only so long before you start thinking seriously about Color Therapy and psychiatrists for your pets.

Meanwhile, the rest of the country is still looking toward California for the next big trend. Judging by the success of "Beverly Hills 90210" and women's ugly platform shoes, it won't be long before we will all be driving around looking at billboards for Amphibian Cell Skin treatments and Aural Sound Wave Therapy. All I can say is, if you don't have a car phone, get one.

Cut Rate Lawyer Ads

Doctors are always trying to decide whether or not to advertise. Most of them don't want to, but they know medicine is changing. Advertising may be the only way to stay in business.

For an example we can look to the legal profession. Lawyers have been advertising for years. Their ads have always been marked by good taste.

Take this discreet advertisement from the classified section of a major newspaper: "$89 DIVORCE." That's it, the entire ad. It is printed in bold letters half an inch high, followed by a phone number.

There are a lot of these ads in the classifieds, like "DIVORCE FROM $95. NO PROPERTY, NO CHILDREN," or "DIVORCE $99, BY APPT. OR MAIL." A number of complex legal problems can be handled through the want ads. "D.W.I. DEFENSE, $400" is a common theme. So is "BANKRUPTCY FROM $250," making it cheaper to divorce someone twice than to go broke. The approach must be working, judging by this ad: "NOTHING DOWN, BANKRUPTCY, OVER 20,000 CASES FILED."

Somehow, I can't see doctors taking this approach. What kind of doctor would place an ad like "GALLBLADDER, $295," or "BABIES DELIVERED, $400, NO TWINS"? You have to wonder about anyone who would pick a doctor based on sale prices, knowing they might spend the rest of their life trying to explain that unusual appendix scar ("I know it looks like a map of Scotland, but it was a real bargain.")

Doctors could never hope to match the timeliness of most lawyer ads. Some attorneys are like high school students, and they quickly flock to the latest fads in liability.

When the state Health Department was investigating immunization reactions in children, it couldn't even notify doctors before there

117

were lawyer ads like this: "Did your child ever get shots? Did they cry? They may be entitled to compensation. Call now."

This happened again when the FDA released an unfavorable study on breast implants. Less than 24 hours later the papers were full of ads like, "Breast Implants? Call now." Potential plaintiffs were signed up by lawyers faster than they could appear on "Oprah."

Lawyer advertising has also made it to television, and I'm not just talking about "L.A. Law," which has become the best advertisement that lawyers have ever had. Lawyers on that show are considered role models because they steal from, cheat on and have sex only with each other, rather than the general public.

The real commercials usually come on late at night, after the talk shows are over. Many of these feature the lawyers themselves, reading their lines off cue cards and making stiff movements with their arms. As actors, they make good lawyers.

Like the newspaper ads, the commercials always start with a question: "Have you ever been injured at all anywhere in a car or building and required any kind of medical treatment or bandage?"

Even if, by some chance, the answer is "yes," they never come right out and tell you what to do. They merely want you to "know your rights," which include the right to sue anyone for any goofy reason you can think of—as if anyone in America needed to be reminded of this.

I suspect that commercials for lawyers will soon be hard to tell from all the other ones on TV. "Are you bothered by painful intestinal gas? You may be entitled to compensation." Or maybe like beer commercials, featuring a summer beach scene full of happy, smiling people in bikinis, until one of them falls and sprains an ankle, leaving them no choice but to sue the volleyball manufacturer for negligence.

Not all professions should advertise, and lawyer ads are a pretty clear example of what can go wrong. I think it will be a while before doctors start using advertising as part of their practices. (Except for some plastic surgeons, who are actually closer to lawyers on the evolutionary tree than they are to other doctors.)

Not all lawyers advertise; maybe the ones who don't could convince the others to quit. But lawyer ads most likely will be around until they become a liability themselves, as people start to sue lawyers because of the pain and emotional anguish produced by their ads. I know they make me sick.

If I could only prove it in court, I might have a case.

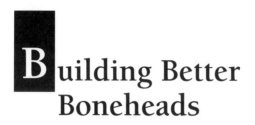

Building Better Boneheads

How to raise a medical ruckus:

Step 1

Think of some bonehead idea. It doesn't matter what it is. In fact, the goofier the better, like saying that gravity causes cancer or that milk is bad for children.

Step 2

Get some quasi-medical fringe group to agree with you. It should have at least one doctor, so it can use "physician" in its name, like "Trustworthy Physicians for Good Responsible Medical Conscience." Never mind that the group also recommends exorcism and bloodletting, as long as its members sound respectable and wear ties.

Step 3

Call a press conference. Have one of the group's members who owns a suit recite the words "milk is bad" approximately 350 times, while mumbling through the part about research to back it up. It also helps to get a famous old doctor with an extensive knowledge of pediatrics (as practiced in 1953), and prop him up next to the table during the presentation.

Step 4

Have the dairy industry issue a backlash statement, along with a 2,000-page research study that would clearly prove something if anyone could read it.

Step 5

Press conference. Make sure that the dairy industry's PR people sound indignant and resentful, like congressmen caught in a bank scandal.

Step 6

Notify the TV doctors. They will do long, thoughtful news pieces that promise to reveal the "true facts." Then they will get the facts slightly wrong, making everyone more confused. The stories consist of interviews with people buying milk at the grocery, along with footage of concerned TV doctors walking down the aisle carrying cartons. After 10 minutes of this, the TV doctor will say, "Evidence shows that there is probably nothing to worry about. Forget we mentioned it."

Step 7

The other doctors will then jump in. They are afraid their patients will make irrational decisions based on inaccurate news stories, like giving their children vodka instead of milk. They feel it is their duty to save them.

Step 8

Press conference. The doctors accidentally say the words "milk is bad" over and over, making sure it is the only thing people will hear: "After checking to see if milk is bad we find that there is probably no evidence that milk is bad, and anyone who says milk is bad should reconsider the evidence in the milk-is-bad controversy."

Step 9

Overwhelming response from people everywhere, universally ignoring the whole thing. People are smarter than fringe groups, TV or doctors give them credit for, and anyone with the common sense that God gave a carrot will give their kids milk once they are a year old.

Still, they can be thankful that in a world knee-deep in dangerous carcinogenic substances, someone is spending time and money worrying about milk.

Severed Arm Still Teaching Students

A few years ago some medical students got into trouble. You might have seen it in the newspaper. It is always news when medical students get into trouble, because it doesn't happen very often.

Somehow it was discovered that these students had been keeping a preserved human arm in their fraternity house.

The arm, which was normally kept in a glass jar on a library table, was spotted on a window ledge by someone walking by, who reported the unusual sight to university police. After some "discussions" with university officials, the arm was turned over to the medical school for safekeeping.

To me, this was an amazing story. Not that medical students would do such a thing—that doesn't surprise me. The amazing thing was that when one of the deans of the medical school was asked about the incident, she said that school officials knew nothing about the arm.

I went to that same medical school, and I knew about it. So did all my friends. One of them mentioned it to me one day as we walked past the house.

"You know, they've got an arm in there," he told me. "I saw it at a party. They keep it in the den."

"Oh," I replied, and we kept walking. If I had been 11 years old, it would have made a great campfire story, but at the time it was only mildly interesting, if a little weird. Remember, we were medical students. We were starting to get used to stuff like that.

I never even wondered how the arm had gotten into the library. Thinking about it now, I can imagine what might have happened. Studying late one night, anatomy final exams coming closer, some poor student must have wanted a few more desperate hours to cram for the test. With the lab closing, he had only one choice: to bring his work home with him. Maybe he even got an "A" in "arm" for that term.

That was over 60 years ago, according to a fraternity spokesman. Since then, the students had grown accustomed to the limb.

Oh, they probably made a few jokes at first ("give me a hand in the library," that sort of thing), but eventually things settled down to a routine, and life went on. The arm became a part of "Phi Chi lore," whatever that is.

In some ways, it makes perfect sense. Medical fraternities, like the 95-year-old arm itself, are relics from the past. They might have once been part of a proud Greek tradition of campus social clubs, but now they are mostly just places to sleep between labs and lectures. I don't know how anyone in medical school could have time for the kind of campus high jinks that characterize most fraternities.

On the other hand, it is hard to imagine this kind of thing happening at any other school.

Medical school can be very dehumanizing, a process that begins with human anatomy class. Each semester the instructors ask for a few minutes of silence for those who gave their bodies in the cause of learning. Over the following weeks the students explore those bodies in every tiniest detail.

It's easy to see how an arm can become just a collection of muscles, arteries and nerves. You forget that it might have once thrown a football or held a loved one, or that it was ever a part of a person at all.

And in fact, that is what must have happened with the arm. The students forgot to show their respect. It would still be resting quietly and semisecretly on their library shelf if only they had not stuck it in the window.

College students have been known to stick other parts of anatomy out of dormitory windows when the warmer weather finally comes, but this must have been a shocking spectacle, even for spring break.

Of course, when confronted, the students did the right thing. Medical students today are much more sensitive than they were 60 years ago.

124

Doctors back then were told that it was more efficient to refer to hospital patients by their room numbers, as in "Nurse, 356 needs his medicine." Nowadays we are taught to consider the whole patient, not just the illness.

After all, these students were not the ones who put the arm into the library, they were the ones who gave it back. Maybe they even learned a bit about respect and dignity in the bargain. Maybe that means they'll be better doctors someday.

Even 60 years later, that arm is still teaching something to medical students. I'm sure that's a legacy the original owner never imagined.

Why Not Medical School?

Every spring college students everywhere are making important choices that will affect their entire lives. Many of them, thanks to several nights of long, hard studying (scattered randomly over four years), will be graduating.

As these people get ready to face the harsh realities of adult life, I want to bring up one option they might not have considered: What about medical school?

Why medical school? For one thing, it is one of the best ways to become a doctor. A mail-order medical diploma might seem attractive, costing less than a single anatomy text and arriving in four weeks, instead of four years. Still, these borderline professional degrees can only lead to embarrassment when facing the harsh scrutiny of malpractice suits or tough medical questions from your relatives over dinner.

To most people, medical school means dissecting dead bodies and memorizing the names of all 203 bones, in between required classes on golf and bad penmanship. This is just not true. Bad penmanship is an elective.

Only medical school gives you a chance to learn gobs of useful information about the human body. Many medical students later put this information to good use by taking care of sick people, but this is only one benefit.

Even if they never practice, medical students have the advantage of constant, continual medical attention for their own bodies. They will always know how to treat their own various aches and pains, which generally means taking a couple of aspirin. They will also be able to spot more serious problems, knowing when aspirin alone is not enough, and when to switch to aspirin plus cold and sinus medicine instead.

Why not medical school? Here are some answers provided by students at a local junior high school when I gave them a boring speech about medicine as a career. Let's examine their concerns one by one, as a guidance counselor would:

"It takes too long"

Unless you are Doogie Howser, medical school takes four years, slightly longer if you recklessly spend time with family or take bathroom breaks. Still, in four years you will be four years older, whether or not you go to medical school, and at least this way you will have thousands of dollars of debt to show for it.

"It's gross"

Parts of it are gross, but this kind of whining means nothing coming from teenagers who routinely sit through "Nightmare On Elm Street" movies while making out in the back row. Besides, nothing I ever saw in medical school prepared me for watching an average "Metallica" video on MTV.

"You have to be a geek"

Of course. What else would you call someone who learns the names of tiny nerve endings, or memorizes elaborate diagrams of biochemical pathways? Medical students are dweebs, but that doesn't mean you have to be a dweeb to apply. Medical school will turn you into one anyway. Many of these people can later be rehabilitated, going on to lead full, productive lives, despite occasional flashbacks of gross anatomy lab.

"But we don't want to be doctors"

Kids today—I just can't relate to them.

I wanted to go to medical school because I wanted to help people, providing health care and humanitarian aid while bringing world peace to all the citizens of Earth. That's what I put in the "personal statement" of my application.

Actually, what I remember is watching episodes of "M#A#S#H" and wanting to be like those zany TV doctors Hawkeye and Trapper, who were always having a great time even though other cast members were routinely being shot or killed in plane crashes. This looks bad on a medical school application, even though the people reading them secretly want to be TV doctors too.

Even without these role models, there are lots of other reasons a medical school education can come in handy. Imagine watching vague TV commercials for medical or personal hygiene products and knowing exactly what they are trying to sell. Or calling your own insurance company to find out why it refused coverage for an "upper respiratory rhinoviral infection" (a cold). Imagine talking to your own doctors and being able to *understand what they are telling you.*

This may be the ultimate health care reform package, where everyone learns the things doctors know. Although details of the plan are not worked out, it is likely that everyone will still be guaranteed access to themselves, unless Senate Republicans manage to eliminate this benefit. There is no better protection for yourself or your loved ones than to learn everything you can about health and medicine now, to avoid the rush.

So forget about that MBA or advanced engineering degree, and call your local medical school instead. Only medical school can give you all the benefits of a medical education, while giving you four more years as a student, safe from the outside world.

It's either that or graduate. Call today.

1-900-DOCTORS

Maybe I'm a little paranoid, but I get worried whenever anyone tries to turn medicine into something like a dial-a-date service. That's what's happening in New York, where they have a new "1-900" number for a service called "Doctors by Phone."

Well, that's just New York, you might say, and so far you would be right. Still, it can't be very long before the idea spreads to other area codes, offering medicine-by-phone to other parts of the country and, at $2 a minute, making trips to the doctor's office obsolete.

You have to wonder about a business that puts people's health on the same level as their daily horoscopes or soap-opera updates.

Even with a real doctor on the other end of the line, relying on the telephone for your medical care is a bit risky, to say the least. No one can really give medical diagnoses or treatment over the phone. They can only dispense the kind of general information found in the "Reader's Digest Home Medical Encyclopedia." This may be useful for someone writing a school report or trying to win an argument, but anyone who wants real help is going to be disappointed.

"1-900" numbers in general are sort of misleading. Late night TV ads are full of beautiful young women who seem desperate for someone to call them at "1-900-LovLine," but there is no guarantee that these same women will be the ones who answer. All you can be sure of is the bill.

The "Phone Doctors" are like that too. Callers have no idea who these doctors are. You would like to believe they are not the same people who were doing phone sales for aluminum siding companies last month, but you can't be sure.

Of course, the doctors have no idea who the caller is either, but this kind of anonymity might appeal to some people. After all, there are some things you just can't ask your regular doctor. Over the phone you can say anything, no matter how embarrassing, without making up some story like, "A friend of mine has this problem . . . "

Despite the risks, the "1-900-DOCTORS" line is catching on, at least in New York. People seem ready to pay for instant access to doctors, whether or not the advice is any good. Soon the phone doctors will have to make some of the same changes that have occurred in other, more traditional branches of medicine.

Like specializing, for one. With more people on the lines, they will have to find some way to sort them out, maybe even one of those irritating voice-mail systems like the banks have: "To speak to a cardiologist, press '2.' For an allergist, press '3.' For a plastic surgeon, press the star. For a nutritionist, press the pound sign. For a psychiatrist, press any two or three numbers at the same time."

You can bet that the regular office-based doctors are going to be upset by this, especially when their patients start using the phone in their lobby to call for a second opinion. After all, they have been taking phone calls from patients for years, often in the middle of the night and usually for free.

They will certainly want a piece of the action. The next time you call your doctor for an appointment, you'd better have your credit card ready. If you thought it was frustrating before, wait until you are put on "hold" at $2 per minute.

Of course, this will only provoke the Phone Doctors, forcing them to take the next step in medical telemarketing. I suppose they will start going through the phone book and calling people at random, during dinner, to ask them if they need any medical advice. "We're having a special on liver diseases and cuticle care," they'll tell them.

"No? How about your horoscope? Aluminum siding?

"OK, forget all that other stuff. Have I got a date for you. . . ."

Multiplication Lessons

In 1994, Vice President Gore attended an international conference on population, where the message was clear: Enough already with the population.

Scientists at this conference were worried that the earth is running out of room. While people in this country have started showing some restraint, it turns out that much of the world is still in the back seat of a '67 Chevy parked in the last row of the drive-in, with only —2— minutes till showtime.

Because of this, many people wonder why so many recent developments have been made in reproductive medicine, particularly because it is a field dedicated to the idea of someday making babies out of thin air. This discrepancy came to light last year when a 62 year-old woman traveled to Italy and, in a startling break from accepted tradition and a clear challenge to the laws of God and humanity, ordered a pizza—*with pineapple*. Afterward, she stopped by an all-night drive-through fertility clinic, becoming the oldest mother since Elizabeth Taylor adopted Michael Jackson.

And this was just one case. Even as the population has burgeoned, Doctors around the world have been discovering many new ways for people to get pregnant, many of them improvements over the older, stickier ways that only sometimes work.

In the simplest cases, the doctor often provides a set of charts and graphs, teaching couples to time their attempts for the best possible chance of conception. This brings to the reproductive process all the spontaneity and romance of a presidential motorcade, proving that doctors can make even sex seem tedious. If this doesn't work, then artificial insemination is used. This eliminates sex altogether, mechanically introducing the egg and sperm together under more favorable conditions, using soft lighting and Julio Iglesias recordings. Next come hormone injections that are so powerful they can even induce ovulation in the person giving the shot.

If there is still no success, then the real scientists take over, using a technique called "In Vitro Fertilization." This procedure allows an egg and sperm cell to come together in the ideal environment, namely a glass specimen dish on a laboratory shelf. It also minimizes the involvement of prospective parents, who might not even be in the same state, and who at this point are pretty tired of the whole thing.

Because the process generally uses an egg donated by a third party, parents could theoretically select the color, size, and style of their new addition, much like picking out a new car. While some people worry about creating "designer children," it is important to remember that any child conceived through this process, no matter what color, shape, or heritage, is probably going to be rich. Otherwise, their parents could never afford the procedure, which costs $15,000-20,000 for each attempt, with only a 1-in-5 chance of success. And no one ever buys just one lottery ticket.

To make things even more unsettling, fertility researchers have even developed a way to get donor eggs from the ovaries of aborted fetuses. They have no plans to try this with humans, at least not until they are able to dig a rescue tunnel through the hate mail from right-to-life groups, who, as comedian Dennis Miller says, will even picket the airlines over an aborted takeoff.

Using this new technique, it would be possible to have a baby who's mother was never born, almost as bad as having the mother turn out to be Nancy Reagan. A child could be younger than his own nephew, making their children third cousins twice removed and, in effect, becoming his own grandparent, giving himself a quarter every time he passes a mirror.

This comes very close to the actual heart of this issue, the thing that has people really worried, which is the possibility of cloning human beings. Almost everyone agrees that cloning would be bad, as demonstrated in countless low-budget sci-fi movies and the docudrama *Jurassic Park*, which showed how a handful of scientists and businessmen were able to develop a secret process for cloning money, raking in billions even before the video sales.

This will be the next big controversy. With cloning, everyone will be able to have all the children they want, allowing humans to procreate randomly without conscious thought or even dating. It could very well disrupt the central, driving force for all life on the planet, besides making it impossible for Little Tikes to keep up with the demand for those little red plastic cars with the yellow tops.

Which Vice President Gore should be certain to bring up at the next population conference, if he can only break through the Vatican's continuing refusal to accept the use of brightly colored riding toys.

The Verdict on Jury Duty

I don't have any important medical news to report at this time because I've been on jury duty, performing my civic responsibility to protect the rights of every American to take public transportation.

That's how everyone in my group got downtown. We happened to be summoned during the coldest period ever recorded in a place without free-roaming polar bears, and no one wanted to risk leaving a car in a frozen tundra. We could have been the first group of jurors ever excused for "hat hair."

Our duty began when we were gathered together in a holding pen (called the "pool," the last place I want to be when it's 24 below) somewhere beneath the Government Center.

There each potential juror was assigned a number and a bar code, which the jury deputies use to scan them in each morning like a can of peaches.

We had a great deputy, and I'm not saying that just because his computer could easily assign me to jury duty again next month. He told us that jurors are picked by random selection, although he himself has never been randomly selected. No one would ever be called again so soon, unless of course there was some sort of computer breakdown.

We were then herded like sheep to an auditorium, which contained—I swear—a piano, probably to help us sing the official jury song.

They showed us an orientation video featuring people who were extremely happy to be on jury duty. These people had obviously built their lives around the chance of someday being jurors, they were now so excited they were having trouble staying in their chairs.

The movie contained a reenactment of an actual trial, but with the boring parts edited out. As a result, the entire thing went from opening to verdict in about 3 minutes. We all figured to be done around lunch.

Next we received instructions on how to be good jury members. Most of these rules were contained in the official "Handbook For Jury Duty." It contained such important tips as no sleeping, no discussing cases with judges, lawyers, defendants, other jurors, friends, family or household pets, and a reminder to keep all personal belongings with you at all times—the courts are evidently full of criminals.

It also included the very important "no playing amateur detective" rule, or the "anti-Mannix" provision. This prohibits jurors involved in trials for brutal, violent crimes from going to the crime scene alone, at night, and "asking around."

Finally, we were ready to begin the main job of jury duty: waiting.

The wheels of justice turn slowly, plus they take long lunch breaks. Everyone waits in the pool, except for bathroom trips, until someone needs a fresh supply of jurors. Depending on the nature of the crime, the deputy then assembles a six- or a 12-pack, along with a few spares in case one of them is defective, and sends them upstairs to the court room.

Until then you wait, sometimes for days. You read, you chat; eventually you begin to hallucinate, imagining yourself as a prisoner of war. You plan elaborate escapes, passing notes to other jurors in the bathroom. Anyone called to the jury office is obviously a spy, and the rest of you work together to hide their hat and gloves.

This goes on until you are called upstairs yourself, where the jury selection process begins.

The most important part of selecting a jury is to carefully weed out anyone who might have some idea what is going on. For example, a case might involve someone who tripped and fell, suffering serious injuries that, although completely invisible to everyone else, might win them a large cash settlement. Naturally, in this case it would be important to eliminate anyone who had any special knowledge or belief in the existence of gravity.

As a doctor, I would also be excluded, even though five or six other doctors might be hired to testify. Having a doctor on the jury could mean a net savings for the court, providing it with a medical person and a jury member in one. After all, it was already paying me $15 a day anyway.

Lawyers do not agree, and so I was kicked off every time. The judges were very considerate, helping me deal with my feelings of rejection. One of them actually said, "Judge not lest ye be judged," which takes on a whole new meaning coming from a professional.

And so I was thrown back into the pool, where I swam around until I was called again, and dumped again, until my jury duty was over. I came away with a much deeper understanding of our legal system and where to have lunch downtown.

It was also reassuring to see that many people are willing to do their civic duty. It made me feel lucky to live in a place that has such a great system of criminal justice, along with a good program of regular computer maintenance.

AMA Follies

With health reform causing enormous changes on the medical scene, the AMA is wasting no time in calling for bold new initiatives into the area of doctor penmanship.

As most people know, the AMA, which stands for American Medical Association, is an Association of Medical Americans who get together once a year in order to issue press statements that make all doctors look greedy, foolish, and self-serving.

Of course, I could be wrong. I am not a member of the AMA myself. There are a lot of doctors who don't belong to the AMA. Some think it is an elitist group that only cares about making money. Others, like myself, refuse to join any group that doesn't have a secret decoder ring.

Because of this, I don't really have any idea what goes on at these AMA meetings until I see the latest goofy headline in the paper, like "AMA Decries Use of Plastic Spatulas," or "Doctors Worried About Increase in Planetary Tilt." For all I know, these reports might have come from doctors who are Ph.D.s in paranormal psychology, or even from people whose last name happens to be "Doctor." I know more about the ADA, the American Dental Association, mostly because I see their stamp on tubes of toothpaste, certifying it as an effective decay-preventing dentifrice.

This year's annual meeting was in June, and instead of focusing on distractions like skyrocketing medical costs or universal health care, the AMA released a hard-hitting statement alerting the public to the fact that doctors have bad handwriting. This makes me wonder if AMA really stands for "Accurate Manuscript Authority." Sloppy handwriting can sometimes cause prescription errors, they said, which can lead to longer hospital stays, or even to illness and death, which can be worse.

Instead of telling them to shape up, they recommended that doctors with poor handwriting (i.e., all of them) type their prescriptions or use a computer. This would work except that doctors can't type and are, for the most part, afraid of computers.

And that's not all. The meeting also produced official AMA pronouncements on several other crucial medical issues, like movie ratings.

Doctors in the AMA, the "Amateur Movie Advisers," are calling for a new, more extensive movie rating system. They want warnings that specifically describe any violent acts. The suggested warning for *Home Alone 2* fills up most of a page, with such listings as "contains scenes of a young boy dropping bricks on a man's head." This could lead to cases where it takes longer to read the warning than to see the movie. The warnings for the *Terminator* movies would have easily filled a three-volume boxed set.

While these goals are certainly worthwhile—I have always been pro-penmanship and anti-Macaulay Culkin—their recommendations for achieving them seem pretty silly, although not as ridiculous as their official stand on breast implants.

For over a year now the AMA has been battling the FDA over the ban on breast implants. The AMA ("Augmented Mammary Advocates") wants them back on the market. Dr. David Kessler, head of the FDA, calls their request "insupportable," citing mountains of evidence linking silicone implants to severe scarring and autoimmune disease, not to mention several multimillion-dollar settlements.

The idea of doctors fighting with the FDA is bizarre and a little scary. No sensible doctor would prescribe any medicine that was banned as possibly dangerous, especially one that provides only cosmetic benefits. I can think of only one reason why some surgeons would continue to use these devices in their patients, at well over $3,000 per operation.

All this is not to say that the AMA has been ignoring health reform altogether. After years of opposing any sort of reform, they finally agreed to support President Clinton's plan, although they reserved the right to send letters to members calling it "the end of life as we know it."

Even so, they quickly went back on their promise. Now, like every junior-grade member of Congress from a state with more than 300 people, they have released their own version of health reform, which protects the interests of insurance companies, specialty groups and the salaries of doctors everywhere. Maybe AMA really stands for "Accumulating Monetary Assets."

The meeting also produced a new AMA plan for dealing with this burning issue of doctor salaries. From now on, when they release figures showing doctor's average salaries, the AMA will include the salaries of interns and doctors in training. Interns are doctors just out of medical school who work about 120 hours a week, at an average wage of about $1.69 an hour. This works out fine because their entertainment expenses consist of sleeping and making an occasional visit home to see their children.

Averaging in the interns will help balance out radiologists, who have become the highest-paid doctors without touching actual patients. Next year I expect the AMA to start including annual salary figures for future doctors still in elementary school.

It is a little-known fact outside of medical circles, but "AMA" means something different to anyone working in a hospital. When patients refuse medical care and demand to leave against their doctor's orders they are said to sign out a.m.a., which stands for "against medical advice."

It's surprising how often that definition might apply out here in the real world as well.

That's Entertainment?

Medical subjects show up all the time in the entertainment field. People love stories about serious diseases and the doctors who treat them, as long as the stories are about someone else.

As a newspaper columnist, it is my job to weed out the sensational, outrageous medical stories from the actual, true, technically correct information. Then I write about the juicy stuff.

This approach allows me to write columns that are just barely related to medicine, and lets me go to the movies and call it "work."

"Cyst," the Mini-Series

(NOTE: This column started a bragging war among local surgeons, with several writing to me with stories about even bigger cysts they had removed. Fortunately, no one sent photos.)

I don't know about you, but my life has certainly been different since the cyst.

It was all I heard about when the story first broke. There, buried on page 10A of the newspaper, was a small, two-column headline: "Doctors remove 180-pound cyst." The story told how doctors at Johns Hopkins Hospital had removed a huge cyst from a woman's abdomen during a 10-hour operation. Details were few, but one fact was clear: This was one big cyst. The patient was not identified. In fact, the doctors could not even discuss the weight of the woman without permission, although they evidently felt at liberty to discuss her cyst once it was removed from her body.

The only person named in the article was a doctor at another hospital in a different state. He said this kind of thing was "abnormally, abnormally abnormal." This "triple-abnormal" statement breaks several rules of grammar and tends to cancel itself out, but I know what he meant.

This article quickly became the talk of our hospital. That morning I came up behind two surgeons in the doctor's lounge and heard them talking about the cyst.

"What? How big? One-EIGHTY? I don't believe it."

"It's true. It was in the paper."

"How much did the patient weigh?"

"They didn't say."

Obviously, doctors are just as interested in gossip as everyone else, although their tastes tend to run a bit to the grotesque. Instead of discussing the new Madonna video or Cher's latest tattoo, they ask each other things like, "What type of incision and approach?" and "How much blood loss? Did they use a laser?" It is just another way to unwind after a busy day in the operating room.

By that afternoon the story of the cyst had spread. I even began to hear details that weren't covered in the original article. "Yes, it had been growing for years," I overheard someone say. "They had to fly the cyst to the Mayo Clinic before they could cut it open." People clearly wanted more details, even if they had to make them up.

It was probably to end this kind of wild speculation that the second story appeared a week later: "Removing massive cyst an ordeal for doctors, patient." This story was longer and more clinical in tone—a cross between the *New England Journal* and "News of the Weird," but the point was still the same: This was some cyst.

More details were given. The operation required some 20 doctors. The cyst was nearly 3 feet across. The weight of the patient was finally revealed, as if it were a big secret that any body harboring a 180-pound cyst must be rather "large-boned" to begin with.

Well, there's no denying the facts: It was one big cyst. Still, the most amazing thing was that the story was in the paper at all.

It's hard to determine exactly when a medical story becomes a popular news item. How do the newspapers find out when something like this takes place in a closed operating room? It's hard to imagine that the doctors might have called the tip to reporters.

A surgeon might mention an 8-pound cyst to a colleague while changing clothes in the locker room. Word of an 18-pounder might make the rounds through the hospital staff, the nurses, and maybe even some of the other patients. But 180 pounds? It would sound too much like bragging, and nobody would believe it anyway.

And besides, if the woman had not given her permission, how could her doctors be outside the room telling the story to the Associated Press? What happened to patient confidentiality? Did this woman want to be famous that badly?

Things have quieted down, but I'm not sure we have heard the last from the cyst. I wouldn't be surprised if more stories appeared, spreading to the other media as well: "Weight loss through massive cyst surgery, on the next 'Oprah.' " This wave of publicity could trigger a flood of patients into Johns Hopkins to have large, heavy portions of their bodies removed.

I wonder if the woman gave up her rights to the story along with the cyst. Can she still sell her story to TV? Every network has loaded their schedules with real-life "docudramas," and the words "based on a true story" are repeated as often as the commercials. With three or four of these made-for-TV movies on each week, the networks are bound to run out of true-life murder-rape-double-suicide plots soon. The story of the cyst is perfect for sweeps week.

Who knows? "Cyst," the miniseries, starring Jaclyn Smith as the woman betrayed by her own body, determined to separate herself from her past." I can see Richard Chamberlain as the dedicated, caring surgeon, trying desperately to save her life and lower her weight, and Ed Asner as the crusty old specialist who sacrifices his own life trying to get the cyst off the table. I think some former child star could play the cyst.

I know, it sounds a little far-fetched. But here's the scary part: The networks won't think so.

A Ride on the Wild Side

I love the State Fair. I love the corn dogs, cheese curds, mini donuts, sno-cones, and, like anyone over age fourteen, the sheer excitement of throwing it all back up on the tilt-a-whirl.

Like many adults, I have a hard time with carnival rides. It wasn't always this way. As a kid I went on rides all the time, the faster and more dangerous the better. I loved feeling my eyeballs rattling around in their sockets, my brain losing its blood supply, and all my viscera being forced into one side of my body. The only time I ever got off a ride voluntarily was when they stopped the Ferris wheel because Laura Solmonsen (not her real name, which was "Lisa") wet her pants while sitting next to me.

This changed as I got older. By high school I starting feeling a little queasy whenever my body was hurled through the air at high speed. The sensation got worse until a few years ago, when I went on a State Fair ride consisting of an enormous salad spinner with a floor that suddenly dropped away, leaving you pinned to the wall like a helpless bug.

I was in medical school at the time, and my training told me I was experiencing a complex physiological process leading up to an embarrassing event—let's call it a *wombat*, using standard medical terminology of cute-sounding animal names for disgusting bodily functions—which would require me to become reacquainted with the food I had eaten that day.

Ever since then, I have had trouble going on rides. Other adults tell me the same thing, leading me to believe there must be some medical reason behind this. As a medical professional, I had no idea what it was, although my experience told me that it probably had a long Latin name.

This is why I own textbooks. Motion sickness, according to one

145

particularly heavy text, is caused by "excessive stimulation of the vestibular apparatus of the ear, which transmits impulses to the cerebral cortex and cerebellum." These impulses go crazy when the visual clues don't match the feelings in the semi-circular canals—or, put simply, Mr. Eye tells a big fib to Mr. Ear, who is desperately trying to figure out where you are in space compared to Mr. Ground.

Unfortunately, the book made no mention of why things get worse when you get older. I assume it is the same thing that happens to all of our body parts. Based on my knees, this would mean that the vestibular apparatus starts to swell up and make crunching noises whenever you use it too much.

Like many people approaching forty, I spend a lot of my time trying to prove I'm not, and this year I decided to prove that my vestibular system was just fine. Some people buy sports cars, some have plastic surgery, but for me, there was only one answer: ride the wild ride.

I was at the fair on opening day before the cows were milked. Asking for advice from some guys with tattoos, I checked out the most frightening rides. These attractions always have names like "The Annihilator" or "The Piledriver"—in fact, the more horrible the name, the longer the line, making you wonder how long people would wait for a ride called "The Disemboweler" or "The Vasectomizer."

The tattoo guys agreed that one ride was the worst, and not just because they were the ones who assembled it and knew how many parts were left over. There was one ride that would prove I had what it takes: the Typhoon.

This was a ride that even men with tattoos avoided. It spins you around while rotating as it revolves, and then it goes backwards. It was the only ride with a "puree" speed. It went so fast people came out younger. The "YOU MUST BE THIS TALL" sign was set at six feet.

Luckily, I was ready. My books listed several ways to combat motion sickness, and I had done my homework. I took Benadryl. I drank fluids, downing two "Big Gulps" on the way over—a volume of liquid capable of supporting its own food chain. I had a motion

146

sickness patch ready to place behind my ear, which reduces the nausea, replacing it with side effects like dry mouth, blurry vision, and urinary retention (probably good considering the big gulps).

I laughed nervously as I climbed aboard. The operator closed the safety bar, a thin metal strip like a curtain rod. This won't save you, but it does allow them to easily locate your body.

With a lurch forward, the ride started.

Despite my curtain rod, was not a single moment during the ride that I was able to positively locate my body. I might have enjoyed it at twelve, but at 38 it was all I could do to keep all my organs inside the car. I tried to focus on the ground, but all I could think of was my stomach and the face of "Lisa" (actually Louise) Solmonsen. I wish she could have been there. Maybe they would have stopped the ride.

Afterward I made my way back to the nice, safe dairy building. There I focused on photos of cows until my stomach started to feel better. Modern Medicine, I realize, can only do so much. I now gladly accept the onset of middle age. After all, there are worse feelings than sore knees.

I also promised myself that, from now on, the most dangerous thing I do at the fair will be eating French fries.

Enquiring Minds Need Therapy

I'm getting tired of being in the dark about the latest medical advances. I guess it's my own fault. All I ever read are textbooks and the latest medical journals.

What I should be reading are the publications sold at supermarket checkout counters, like the *National Examiner*. How else would I know that it is now possible to reverse the natural aging process, or that people can now perform their own liver transplants in the privacy of their homes?

Such startling medical reports might surprise anyone who thinks these publications are full of ridiculous stories about bizarre religious cults and space alien babies. (Actually, the space aliens are only flirting with us, as revealed in a story about giant sex symbols carved into a field in Peru. Evidently, humans are not the only ones who have trouble making commitments.)

Medical news makes up a large part of the *Examiner*. It even has a medical page, called "Medical News You Can Use," and it is just chock-full of late-breaking medical research. Take a look at some of these recent scoops:

Women can now prevent osteoporosis by using a nasal spray made from extract of fish heads.

Losing teeth? No problem, now that dentists can easily replace them with small pieces of sea coral.

WARNING! Nutra-Sweet can cause seizures in children with seizure disorders, who already had seizures anyway.

There is no longer any need for painful and expensive plastic surgery, thanks to an exciting new "accupressure face-lift" technique, which took years off Melanie Griffith.

Like most things you read in these papers, there is a grain of truth behind each of these stories (except for Melanie Griffith, who does not actually exist outside of the popular press). In most cases that grain has been bloated and hideously distorted, much like the picture of Liz Taylor on the cover, but a tiny fragment of the truth remains. This allows papers like the *Examiner* to present new medical breakthroughs, along with their extensive coverage of fertility problems in former Charlie's Angels.

In this way readers can stay medically informed while still enjoying themselves. Most medical journals are not much fun, being full of dreary references and footnotes. They hardly ever feature diet plans of soap opera stars. Medical reporters have to be careful to document every step of their research, and spend hours checking their facts before going to press; the reporters at the *Examiner* spend their time pasting new heads on celebrity photos. Besides, medical textbooks cost a hundred dollars; the *Examiner* goes for 99 cents. You can see which one is going to appeal to the casual reader.

Some say that no one really believes these stories, unless they also believe the ones about the sexy space aliens, in which case they probably need more than a medical doctor. Let's hope they're right. Still, a lot of people are buying them. The circulation of the *National Examiner* is over 2 million, and only some of those people are wearing foil inside their hats to block out transmissions from space.

The others are people just like you and me, only they are going to run into trouble the next time they visit a doctor and ask for the new miracle zinc injection that will completely erase all disease in their body.

Of course, if I become a regular *Examiner* reader I'll know what the heck they're talking about. The only hard part will be getting the latest copy without feeling like a total idiot. It probably means weekly trips to the supermarket, in disguise, where I can secretly throw one into my cart along with some animal crackers at the check-out counter.

It will be worth it, especially after I receive my "Ginko Biloba" cream, which, as regular *Examiner* readers know, is "an ancient Chinese remedy that helps reverse the body's aging process." I can't wait. I'll have to be careful not to use too much and send myself back to childhood, or worse, back to fetus stage. Otherwise, I'll end up as a headline in a future issue: "Practicing Doctor, Only THREE DAYS OLD, Warns Of Misleading Medical Tabloids. Claims not to be Space Alien Baby."

I hope they at least let me keep my original head.

Batman and Mental Illness

I get excited every time a new *Batman* movie opens. I'm sure anyone interested in the workings of the human mind would feel the same way.

A lot of people think that these movies are just comic book stories on the big screen. They are wrong. These movies are important to doctors because of the deep psychological undercurrent that has always been a part of the Batman legend.

Batman is not your average hero. This is the story of a man, Bruce Wayne, who saw his parents murdered before his eyes, a scene so monstrous that it warped his mind forever. Because of these psychic scars he was somehow able to convince himself that it was a good idea to dress up in a bat suit and hunt down criminals.

And Batman is one of the saner people in these movies.

Like most medical students, I worked in mental health facilities and locked psychiatric wards as part of my training. We were supposed to learn more about mental illness, but when we finished the rotation (at least, those of us who were free to leave) we had seen little in the way of interesting psychiatric pathology. Everybody there seemed pretty normal.

The characters in *Batman* movies are different. Here are some of the more interesting case reports from the most recent movie:

Case Number 1

"Batman," (not his real name), the hero in the black suit. This is not a man who is flying with both wings in the air.

151

Case Number 2

The villain, the "Penguin," a short, demented bird fancier in formal attire. The Penguin may have once been merely depressed, but he has come a long way since then. Now he lives in a sewer pipe with thousands of small, flightless waterfowl. He collects umbrellas. He rides a giant rubber ducky. He wants, as they used to say in James Bond movies, "to rule the world."

Case Number 3

"Catwoman," the heroine/villainess, a young woman with an obsessive feline disorder manifesting itself as a bizarre type of schizophrenia. Dressed in skin-tight black vinyl sewn together with cat gut, she plays a game of Bat-and-Mouse with our hero, her emotional state spinning wildly between playful seduction and cold animal ruthlessness. "Balanced" is not a word that applies to Catwoman. She has to be a little crazy just to wear that outfit, which is, as a friend of mine says, "screaming out for a yeast infection."

Not a bad display of abnormal behavioral pathology for a comic book movie. There are clinical psychologists in big-time county hospitals who have never been exposed to anyone half as weird as the people in *Batman Returns*.

And that's just on the screen. Go to one of these openings and take a look around you. These are people who have been just counting the days (maybe the hours or even the minutes) until this movie opened. Try to imagine what kind of material they would make for someone's doctoral thesis. (No fair picking the ones in full Joker makeup—at least make it a challenge.) Many of them will still be sitting there as you get up to leave, quietly waiting for the next show, and the next. Because the thing about *Batman* is this: As crazy as it seems, it could happen. At one time, Bruce Wayne was a normal guy, just like everyone else. All it took was an incredibly horrible episode of wrenching emotional trauma, and it turned him into Batman, the caped crusader. Who can say if any of us would handle things any better?

So you may see me there too, purely for professional reasons, of course. I want to refresh my knowledge of abnormal psychology and brush up on the latest psychiatric trends. I won't be buying any Batman T-shirts, or coffee mugs, or dolls, or glow-in-the-dark Frisbees, or automobile air fresheners. I still have most of that stuff from last time.

But I will go, and I'm sure I'll have fun, watching the crowd as well as the screen. You may see me there. I'll be the one taking notes in the dark.

Paging Dear Abby

You've felt it, haven't you? An underlying uncertainty that makes you question all your decisions and look three or four times before crossing the street. It happens every time Ann and Abby are out of town, leaving us to fend for ourselves.

I don't know how the people in charge of the newspapers can let something like this happen. There is never even any warning, just a notice that appears one day to tell us that for the next two weeks Ann Landers and Abigail Van Buren will be on vacation.

I liked it better when they were feuding. At least they never went on holiday together, leaving us alone and advice-less.

And what do we get instead? "A selection of favorite past letters," sort of Abby and Ann's greatest hits. I didn't know they had favorites; I thought that every letter was equal under the advice columnist's oath. Ann got in trouble for reprinting letters once before, and I can't see how a warning label makes it any more acceptable now.

This old, leftover advice is of no use to people who need help and need it fast. What are they supposed to do? Should they leave their spouses right away or wait until the two weeks are over? Are they going to have to send a thank-you note to the cousin who gave them a set of broken ice-tea glasses for a wedding present? Should they "get counseling?"

It's even harder for the people who wrote the letters that are reprinted. Just when they had gotten their lives in order and put their terrible troubles behind them, "Dear Abby" brings them out of the mothballs and prints them on page 6E for everyone to see. Friends and co-workers are bound to recognize them, and everywhere they go folks will be asking them, "Harold, wasn't this you? I thought you took care of that little problem." High school reunions,

154

divorces, wedding receptions, sleepovers—a lot of water has passed under the bridge since those letters were written. Why bring them up again?

I guess everyone needs to get away, but I hope from now on the twins can work ahead a bit, maybe answer a few extra letters a day until the two weeks are covered. Either that, or go on separate vacations and cover for advice emergencies, like doctors have to do. Sure, it's an awesome responsibility, but it comes with the dated photo at the top of the column: When you are Dear Abby, you need to be there for people.

Michael Jackson's Doctor

I'm sure everyone was relieved to find out that Michael Jackson has an actual disease and is not merely the most eccentric person in the entire history of human behavior.

This fact was revealed in a televised interview with Oprah Winfrey, which was seen by more people than currently own TV sets. Not one to shy away from hard questions, Oprah asked him about his skin color, which has been gradually fading since 1978 and is now about the shade of unpasteurized milk. Michael revealed that this is the result of a rare skin condition that causes his skin to fade, eventually turning him transparent and making him the perfect mate for someone like Lisa Marie Presley.

A prominent Beverly Hills dermatologist confirmed the diagnosis at a press conference the next day. According to his doctor, Jackson does indeed have vitiligo, a rare disease that causes people to grab their crotch every 60 seconds.

No, the dermatologist explained that vitiligo actually destroys the pigment cells that give skin its color. Treatment is limited to makeup, which most people use to darken the vitiligo spots. Michael, showing the trend-setting style for which he is famous, uses makeup instead on the rest of his skin to make it match the diseased areas. (The mascara and lipstick are a separate problem, having nothing to do with the disease and used only to make him look like a younger, hipper version of the Joker.)

Michael also told Oprah that he had received "very little" plastic surgery. Even while saying this he was careful to keep his head slightly turned to the side. His nose is now so narrow it disappears when viewed straight on, leaving nothing but two large eyes behind a few strands of hair.

Unfortunately, no plastic surgeon was on hand to back this up.

You can understand why Michael's plastic surgeon would be hard to reach, presumably having retired via Learjet to his own private island nation in the Caribbean.

The Michael Jackson case is a milestone in the use of "celebrity doctors," physicians who take care of famous people. Besides all the other problems of dealing with well-known patients, celebrity doctors can find themselves thrust into the spotlight at any moment. They must be willing to go on TV and discuss important celebrity medical problems, despite the very real risk of getting rich from a flood of new referrals.

In the Jackson case, Michael had his doctor make a statement in case anyone doubted the story about the skin disease. In this way, he was able to come up with a medical excuse for his own bizarre behavior. This is the celebrity equivalent of a doctor's note to get out of gym class. Now people will feel sympathy for him instead of openly questioning his racial and species types.

This is bound to trigger a wave of famous-patient case reports in the news, as other celebrity doctors step forward to defend the oddball quirks of their own famous patients.

Some of them are going to have to get even more personal. I assume someone like Madonna has a doctor, although I'm not sure what they could say at a press conference. Has her doctor seen anything that the rest of us haven't? The woman has nothing left to use for shock value. All she can do is release copies of her Pap smears, or maybe enclose her upper GI X-rays with her next album.

In the meantime, medical science has taken some pressure off Michael Jackson. There has been a lot of criticism of Michael's appearance and effeminate manner. Casting some of those doubts aside, he said during the Oprah interview that he was "proud to be a black man." Thanks to the expert opinion of one celebrity doctor, we now know that he really is, at the very least, black.

Year of the Prostate

(WARNING! The following contains information about the prostate gland. Men over 40 who have recently had physical exams should skip ahead to avoid unpleasant flashbacks.)

It is clear that the ancient Chinese astrologers really knew what they were doing when they designated this year as "Year of the Prostate."

Until the end of last year ("Year of the Nasal Septum") you never heard much about prostate glands. Most people, even the half of the population that own them, had no idea what they were for. "Prostate" was just another scary-sounding body part, even more frightening than "cerebellum" or "pyloric sphincter." People knew only that it was located somewhere "down there," close to a lot of important equipment, and must therefore be important too. Many of them were still making the common first-year medical student mistake of saying "prostrate," which is actually what you are after having it checked.

Now, in the Year of the Prostate, the small, troublesome glands are turning up everywhere. People bring them up at dinner parties. Young, hip characters in TV sitcoms talk about their fathers'. In the movie *The Paper*, Robert Duvall goes to a prostate specialist and makes bagel jokes in the newsroom. Public awareness of prostate glands is now at an all-time high.

I first noticed this when I opened a copy of a national newsmagazine during breakfast and found myself facing a large (to me, anyway) full-color diagram of the male reproductive system, including the part that rhymes with Venus. Even with my medical training, I had to quickly flip the page before turning back to my Cheerios.

The diagram was part of an ad for a medicine that is supposed to shrink swollen prostates. The prostate is not a bad gland, it is just in a bad place. It is wrapped around a main section of the male plumbing, which gets pinched off as the gland slowly grows larger over the years. This happens to most men as they get older, and is just a part of life, namely the part where they get up at night to go to the bathroom.

Naturally, all the publicity is making some people even more anxious and fearful about prostates. The best thing for these people to do is call the doctor and set up a prostate exam for their husbands.

This is the procedure where the doctor puts on a single glove, like Michael Jackson, which invariably causes every patient to turn pale and say the same thing: "I hate this part."

This is, of course, the correct response, which allows the doctor to make a little check in the "normal" box on the physical form.

Most men survive the exam itself, even making jokes about it with their friends afterward. Some pretend they have endured some incredibly macho ordeal, like skydiving into an active volcano, which naturally makes their friends want to have theirs checked too. (Women have been having things like this done every year with very little whining, which is just another reason to be glad they are the ones giving birth. Given a choice, many men would simply say "I hate this part," and the human species would never reproduce.)

While few men need medicine, these exams are useful because they also check for signs of prostate cancer. This is the unspoken threat behind all of the uneasy fear and vague advertising. Prostate cancer, not just enlargement, is the real reason for every male over 50 to know what his prostate gland is up to. All the publicity may be spoiling a few breakfasts, but may also be sending men to the doctor, which might accidentally do some good for the wrong reasons.

If not, there is more publicity on the way. Variety magazine recently ran this ad, placed by a well-known talent agency: "Seeking name celebrity with an enlarged, noncancerous prostate to make personal appearances and serve as a paid spokesman for a drug company." Although this agency has been able to find celebrity spokespeople for denture creams and obsessive-compulsive disorder, they are having some trouble finding a suitably famous prostate. This may be more than anyone, even Geraldo Rivera, wants the public to know, particularly when you imagine those personal appearances. (Remember Martha Raye flashing her dentures on TV, and you'll see why I worry.)

In the Year of the Prostate, there soon won't be anyone who doesn't know where their prostate, or that of a loved one, is located. Thanks to intense media coverage, the prostate will soon be just another household gland, causing no more anxiety than the average thyroid or salivary gland.

And then we'll all be ready for next year, designated on the calendar as "Year of the Fallopian Tube." It's only fair.

Flu Shots Increase Ratings

Imagine how hard it has been for poor daytime TV hostess Sarah Purcell since a doctor on a live national broadcast accidently replaced her brain with one from a chipmunk.

I can think of no other explanation. Who else would have agreed to such a bonehead scheme? The quest for more realistic programming has finally led to the idea of giving actual medical care on TV. Because of this, millions of people saw a nervous doctor give Purcell an unneeded flu shot with the same syringe he had just used on her cohost, Gary Collins.

Shortly afterward we began receiving daily updates on blood tests performed on Collins. The first reports were sketchy, telling us only that he is married to a former Miss America, so he must be, you know, OK. Later we learned that his HIV and hepatitis tests were negative. This is very reassuring, although no one saw them actually draw the blood on the air, so you never know.

The TV people must not have realized that doctors don't often give shots; nurses do. The last time I gave a shot was when my sister broke out in hives from a chlorine overdose at a local swimming pool. Before that I'd have to go back to my rotation in a large county hospital, where the medical students did everything short of open-heart surgery. Holding a celebrity arm under hot lights on national television—who can say any doctor would have done better?

Several nurses saw the picture in the paper and told me that not only did he reuse the needle, but it appeared that he also gave the shot in the wrong place and using the wrong technique, going just under the skin instead of deep into the muscle. All in all, Purcell may have been lucky to survive.

Nurses, on the other hand, give shots every day. They are very good at it. The doctor should have known this. He could have made the segment much more realistic by simply signing a chart and then stepping out in the hall, moving on to his next appointment, perhaps a game show, while the nurse did it correctly.

I hope this little incident doesn't put a stop to this exciting new trend in reality TV. I myself have a list of television personalities that I would love to see getting certain medical procedures on the air, and not just vaccinations. I know I would enjoy seeing Bryant Gumble have an arthroscopy, or watching Barbara Walters being scratch-tested for allergies. This could even result in the long-awaited colon cancer screening for Geraldo, which would undoubtedly be a live pay-per-view event.

Meanwhile, we'll have to settle for Gary Collins' latest serum testosterone levels, and hope that next time they pick someone more used to inflicting pain in front of a crowd, like maybe a politician.

Four Letter Word for Football: OUCH

Last Fall, with the leaves threatening to bury the yard, garage, and dog, I decided to spend a Sunday afternoon watching football with my son.

He was only 2, but you could tell the game made a big impression on him. On the very first play he got a worried look on his face, like when he tasted strained beets, and said, "Ouch." He said it again every time somebody got tackled or fell down, which is to say, every single play.

Obviously, he is just a kid. Toddlers cannot appreciate the finer points of football. He can't possibly grasp the level of skill involved, the beauty of the passing attack, or the complexity of the various formations. What he saw was a bunch of grown-ups running into each other, on purpose, and trying to knock each other down.

This made absolutely no sense to him, possibly because of his own recent battles with gravity. It wasn't that long ago that not falling down was a full-time job for him. And we have been telling him for months that pushing people is not OK.

But here were grown men trying viciously to batter each other to the ground, and only getting in trouble when they held on.

I used to like watching football myself. At least, I think I did. I never played because I was too small, or too fat, or too nerdy—I forget the exact reason, but in our high school this meant one thing: dweeb city. People who weren't cool enough to play were supposed to go to games and cheer for those who were. I have watched football ever since, which proves how long high school brainwashing can last.

Before my son said "ouch" I never noticed that every football play ends in 9 or 10 separate brutal collisions. The center hikes the ball and is instantly flattened. The person taking the ball will be

163

tackled, generally by two or three others. Even when the receivers are catching touchdown passes, the linemen are banging into each other like crash-test dummies in a 1972 Vega. The people in "skilled positions" (a sports term meaning white millionaire quarterbacks) are regularly maimed—in fact, some defensive coaches believe that's the point. Worst of all, many players now celebrate particularly cruel or vicious hits, dancing around like M.C. Hammer with bad jock itch. No wonder NFL teams keep trauma surgeons on the sidelines.

You see retired football players on TV all the time, usually sitting in broadcast booths wearing blazers the color of radioactive isotopes. They don't walk around much; some of them can't, having paid for years of gridiron glory in knees and lumbar discs. Most of them are washed up at 30, cut loose from the game with no real skills, unable to go up a flight of stairs without sounding like a bowl of Rice Krispies.

Even with my brainwashing, I know I would never want my son to play football. Luckily, kids today are smarter than I was. A lot of them, even popular ones, go out for sports like soccer, which does not require full body armor and a dental plan. Meanwhile, lots of older, formerly non-cool people are also staying quite active, enjoying sports that keep them healthy for a lifetime. They may never play in a Super Bowl, but they'll still be around to watch them when the roman numerals run out, although they would probably rather go jogging instead.

When the attorney general called for a crackdown on TV violence, everyone assumed she was talking about the endless parade of crimes and murders in prime time. I know a lot of people will call me a Communist pinko wimp crybaby, but I think she should tune in and see what happens on Sunday afternoons.

I tried watching again one Monday night after my son was asleep, but it was no fun. I kept finding myself saying "ouch." I couldn't enjoy the slow-motion replays of fearsome collisions. I couldn't listen to the dull, wet thud of bodies hitting together, amplified by giant satellite dishes that catch every grunt and moan. All I remember was the medical team running out on the field to help an unconscious player, just before the TV announcers cut to a beer commercial.

I think my son was right. After all, he was certainly right about the strained beets.

Wild Pitch at the Movies

It was somewhere in the middle of *The Flintstones* that I realized I was tired of bad movies. I was tired of waiting in line to buy tickets for them, tired of sitting in crowded theaters waiting for them to end, even tired of bringing home videos and finding them half-watched with the tape stopped in the middle, a sure omen of a bad movie.

It was at that point I decided, as I'm sure many of you have done, that I was going to make my own movie.

Theoretically, this would have been slightly easier during Pitch Day, an annual moviemaking event held by a local film group. Each year it brings to town a group of prominent Hollywood producers, inviting writers to "pitch" them ideas for movie scripts. This year, frustrated by bad movies, I decided to sign up.

I knew it was ridiculous to imagine that I could write a great movie. Films like *Field of Dreams* or *Dances With Wolves* require years of dedication, hard work, and Kevin Costner.

Bad movies are different. (In this case, "bad movies" are stupid movies that should not have been stupid, judging by the big-name directors and actors, often Robert De Niro, in the credits. Examples include *Man Trouble*, *Mad Dog and Glory*, and *The Last Action Hero*. This doesn't count films like *Ace Ventura, Pet Detective*, which are stupid on purpose, and sometimes turn out to be good.) If these Hollywood people wanted scripts for bad movies, there was no problem. Anyone should be able to write a bad movie. Some of them (*Toys*) seem to be filmed without any script at all, making you wonder how they knew how many actors to hire.

Someone must have once had high hopes for movies like this. Where did they go wrong? Was it bad writing? Bad acting? Bad directing, bad editing? I had no idea, but I figured it might as well be bad writing, and that's where I come in.

I wasn't completely without script experience, having written the hilarious "fractured humerus" skit for our medical school talent show. Although I had never written an entire movie, I knew there were certain qualities that my script should have, like action, humor, romance, and a main character about my own age, height and body build who could conceivably be played by me. This worked for Sylvester Stallone, resulting directly in *Rocky* and indirectly in *Stop or My Mom Will Shoot!* While I would never leave medicine, I knew it was not impossible to become an internationally known star of action-oriented doctor films in my spare time.

Why not? Hollywood is obviously starved for ideas. Movie theaters have become "Nick at Nite," showing nothing but big-screen versions of old TV sitcoms. Without new ideas we would only be faced with big-budget, all-star remakes of "My Mother the Car" and "F-Troop." (This joke originally used "Gilligan's Island" and "The Brady Bunch," until I learned that these movies are actually in production. Be afraid, be very afraid.)

Armed with this knowledge, along with a magazine article on scriptwriting that included the proper use of the term "babe," I was ready. Only one thing was holding me back: no script. I didn't necessarily consider this a liability. In the worst case, the producers would love my pitch and ask to see the script, whereupon I'd tell them the dog ate it and promise to send it next week. I wasn't a student most of my life for nothing.

Pitch Day finally arrived. We were each assigned to a producer and given 10 minutes to pitch our stories. When it was my turn, I told a story based on my life as a medical student.

Naturally, I doctored it up a bit, liberally sprinkling in elements that never actually happened but that audiences enjoy in movies, like friendship, romance, happiness, and naked people who were not yet dead. I used every ounce of my energy, waving my arms as I wove a cinematic tale of life, love and redemption, the plot unfolding at breakneck speed while my words created images so vivid and emotionally engaging that you could hardly tell I was making it up as I went along.

The producer listened quietly, then offered a few helpful suggestions. The story was fine, she said, but there was a problem with the characters. Unfortunately, the principal character, who was based on myself, was not a believable person. My wife has been saying this for years.

I wasn't the only casualty. This kind of thing happened to a lot of other prospective screenwriters on Pitch Day. The producers talked about things like character, motivation and integrity. They wanted stories that were consistent, interesting and, yes, even meaningful. None of which explains *Sliver, Bad Girls,* or any movie with Madonna.

The question remains: Why all the bad movies? I still don't know, which leaves me with only one thing to do: As painful as it seems, I'm afraid I may have to take another look at *The Flintstones.* This movie stuff is evidently a lot harder than I thought, babe.

Sick Policy

I have been in school most of my life, between high school, college, medical school, internship, and residency. For all I know, I may even have accidently repeated a few grades without my knowledge.

Despite all this advanced learning, I still have no idea what our government is up to, or why large corporations like insurance companies or drug and tobacco manufacturers are allowed to have so much power over normal people. This is as close to a political statement as you will find in this book. Sorry if you weren't able to stay awake. We now return you to the goofy medical jokes.

What's Wrong with Health Insurance

A lot of people are wondering what effect the new administration will have on the crisis in health care. As a trained medical professional, here's my projection of what will happen to health care in this country: I have no idea.

Nobody knows what is going to happen. There are a lot of government economists and health care analysts who have theories, along with charts and diagrams on large computer printouts in four colors of ink, but nobody really knows.

A lot of people are to blame for the current mess, including some doctors, but one big problem is health insurance. It's pretty clear that the experts are going to have to come up with something better than we have now.

I don't have any charts or graphs, but I do work in the health care field, and, if nothing else, I know what is wrong with most medical insurance as it exists today:

It doesn't cover everyone

Insurance companies are very careful about who is covered by their plans. They know it would cost a lot of money if they accidentally accepted anybody who was going to be sick some day.

Except in group plans, insurance companies can refuse anyone for any reason, like spraining an ankle. Anyone wanting insurance has to go through an elaborate screening process, which includes questions like this: "Have you ever had a cold or a sexually transmitted disease? Check Y or N." Nobody can even make it through the questionnaire without developing high blood pressure or other symptoms that make them ineligible.

It covers everyone the same

In most plans, everyone pays the same premium. This is the exact opposite of auto insurance, where they can raise your rates if you so much as happen to witness an accident while driving.

In health insurance, people who smoke and eat pork rinds pay the same rate as marathon runners. Your only reward for taking care of yourself is that you live longer, which allows you to pay more premiums.

It covers everything

HMO plans were supposed to control rising costs, but they overlooked one thing: About 10 percent of their clients are people who really like going to the doctor, even when they are not very sick. Now they can go all the time because they think it is free. It isn't. These people clog up the system so that others can't get in, no matter how sick they are.

It doesn't cover everything

I don't know exactly what my insurance plan covers. Neither do you, unless you have been trapped in your home by a major flood with nothing to read but the cards in your wallet. People often believe they have good insurance, only to find out later that it only covers 80 percent of any takeout food ordered from their hospital room.

Insurance companies know this, and they have taken a simple, straightforward approach to the problem: If you don't know whether a particular service is covered, it isn't.

They are happy to tell you this when you call. Many of them have set up "800" numbers that people can call to be told "no" 24 hours a day.

Some companies use creative ways of saying "no," like promising to reimburse someone for a weight loss program if they manage to keep it off through the holidays, or to pay for their health club membership if they make it to the next Olympics.

171

Others get around saying "no" by saying that any treatment will be paid for if it is ordered by a physician. In my experience, you have as much chance of filling a prescription for a dirigible as you would of getting your insurance to pay for an orthopedic mattress, no matter what your doctor says.

And all insurance companies agree to pay when a doctor recommends a chiropractor if, in the entire history of medicine, this ever actually occurs.

It is run by insurance companies

This is the biggest problem with health insurance. It is run by huge corporations who have nothing to do with health care. They skim 30 percent of all the money right off the top, just for making everyone fill out forms in triplicate.

Obviously, this is a complex subject, full of contradictions. I was hoping to present my five-point plan for completely revitalizing the health care industry, which eliminates insurance companies and asks some doctors to charge less money, but I seem to have run out of room.

Too bad, because it is 100 percent guaranteed to work, and I know insurance companies would be happy to pay for the plan just as soon as it is prescribed by doctors everywhere.

Fear and Broccoli

The last few months of his presidency were certainly rough on George Bush. First there was that Saddam Hussein thing. Then he got violently ill on an important Japanese diplomat. Then his reelection campaign faltered, allowing Bill Clinton to gain crucial momentum and eventually triumph.

Then, on top of everything else, came new scientific evidence that broccoli may be the most potent anticancer agent ever known.

Details of the Johns Hopkins broccoli study were released during the campaign, and the bumpy green vegetable was soon on everyone's lips. News like this travels fast, and most people quickly learned that there is a chemical in broccoli that helps prevent cancer.

Granted, that's not much information to go on. But the statement did feature two very important words, "prevent" and "cancer," next to each other. That alone was enough to set off a wave of broccoli buying like we haven't seen since the oat-bran craze.

Scientists have known for a long time that certain chemicals can stimulate enzymes to protect cells from cancer. In fact, several other substances have been promoted as anticancer "wonder drugs" in the past. Broccoli is different because a) it is not illegal, b) it may actually work, and c) you do not have to travel to Mexico to get it. Broccoli is cheap and plentiful, and a lot of people started stuffing themselves with the tree-like stalks right away.

Which is exactly what anyone must do to get the full benefits of broccoli therapy. Unlike the fat-burning grapefruit pill that is advertised on late-night TV, there is no way put the broccoli chemical into pill form. That means one thing to those who want to reduce their risk: broccoli, and plenty of it.

Obviously, this was bound to have a significant impact on Wall Street broccoli futures. Small farmers, or even suburban dwellers with back-yard gardens, decided to uproot the asparagus and rhubarb in favor of this new cash crop. Chinese restaurants experienced a run on beef and broccoli, and "Broccoli on a Stick" became the hot concession in the food building at State Fairs.

Broccoli chips, broccoli muffins, broccoli ice cream—go ahead, imagine the oddest combination you can think of, and soon you could buy it at the grocery store or local health-food boutique. The specific chemical, "sulforaphane," was added to the list of famous secret ingredients like "retsin" and "hexychlorophene." Broccoli-eating became synonymous with good health. People began commenting on someone's vitality and vigor by saying, "Boy, there's a guy who really eats his broccoli."

And that's when the politicians stepped in. Bush was on record with the whole broccoli thing. "Read my lips," he told us. "No more broccoli." He had no choice but to take a step back on the broccoli issue, decrying his earlier anti-broccolism. Either that or blame someone else, probably Congress.

The other candidates were quick to focus on the "broccoli gap." They wondered out loud, in front of reporters, if the president had the guts to "do what it takes" to prevent cancer. "For all we know he probably also is against fiber," they said, shaking their heads sadly.

Driven by a wave of pro-broccoli sentiment, the voters were swayed. They knew they could never cast their vote for anyone pro-cancer. They remembered the president's words from last year. "I just don't like it," Bush told them then. "Look, I'm the president, and nobody can make me eat broccoli if I don't want to."

I guess at least one of those things is still true.

Hillary Care— She's the Mom

Well, the presidential committee for health care reform finally released its plan, which will guarantee the right of every American citizen to have an apple each and every day, in a concerted, groundbreaking effort to keep the doctor away.

The plan was put together by Hillary Rodham Clinton and about 30,000 expert advisers in the health care field, most of whom are lawyers.

It was a big job, particularly when you consider some recent statistics: Health care is a $60 hepto-gazillion industry in this country. More than $1.37 of every dollar is now spent on health care. The entire GNP during the late '80s was spent on cholesterol testing alone. Just the interest on the portion of the national debt created by spiraling health care costs. Fifty percent.

What all this means is that many people are being forced to go without any health insurance at all. This is fine with them because it means never having to fill out any forms, at least until they get sick. Then they lose everything trying to pay hospital bills which list things like "aspirin (2), $5.78. Cup (1) of water to swallow above, $2.55. Thermomagnetic-nuclear-gizmotronic scan (results: normal), $1—see attached list of zeros."

Many people were surprised that Hillary Clinton was chosen to head such an important committee, but there is a very good reason for this: She is the mom.

Women are always the ones to make important health care decisions for their families. Moms usually select the family doctor and call to make the appointments, even when their husbands are sick. When sensitive, caring, "new age" fathers bring in their children for ear infections, you can bet they are carrying with them a list of questions from their wives.

175

It is Hillary's job to sell the plan to doctors and other health care providers everywhere. The final details were supposed to be released earlier, but that deadline was pushed back several times, largely because of the complexity of coordinating various cost-ratio analysis factors—basically, the dog (or, in this case, the cat) ate the homework.

Most of the plan has now been revealed in top secret reports appearing in newspapers. We are now entering the official rebuttal process, known as the period of Congressional Whining. Here are some highlights of the plan:

Universal access

Everyone will be guaranteed access to a doctor, even if they don't want to go. All Americans will be issued a Universal Health Card, which will also be good in cash machines and finer department stores. If you go over your limit, for example a long hospital stay, someone will be assigned to come to your room and cut up your card.

Malpractice

The lawyers on the committee are going to have to figure out some way to control the ridiculous number of malpractice suits that are crippling the present system. Other lawyers will then sue them for lost compensation and pain and suffering.

Drug prices

Manufacturers will control the cost of current drugs, and must set new drug prices based on reasonable factors, not the latest NFL free-agent negotiations. CEOs of major drug companies who make more than $5 million (there were several last year) will be required to get sick themselves.

Prevention

The committee realizes that a few dollars spent on preventive care can save thousands later. All children would receive immunizations to prevent dangerous, potentially brain-damaging conditions, including vaccines against DPT, MMR and the NRA, with boosters during campaign years.

Specialty care

The new plan relies on primary care doctors, letting them handle simple problems without referring patients to expensive specialists. These specialists have traditionally been paid two or three times what primary doctors make, but, according to a recent survey of doctors, new Medicare rules have started to narrow that gap. Of course, the people doing the survey—this is true—paid specialists $75 to respond, compared with $50 for primary doctors.

Paperwork

Insurance companies now get a third of all the money in the health care system just for making people fill out forms. The new plan would keep things simple, limiting the paperwork to a single, universal claim form for all medical bills. Although the form will probably be in some language other than English, it should be no problem for any qualified lawyer with a working knowledge of social economic theory.

There you have it, the plan so far. It will take several years to phase in these changes, and experts recommend holding off on any serious illness for now.

Still, if it works, everyone in the country will finally have access to competent, dependable medical care. It will be as simple as calling the White House and asking them to make you an appointment. Be sure to ask for Hillary.

Drug Companies Strike Back

Although President Clinton's Health Care Reform package was quickly rejected by Congress, it has already had one obvious effect: The drug companies are fighting back.

According to recent scary government reports, drug companies in this country have been routinely practicing price gouging and dishonest marketing techniques. Manufacturing prescription drugs has become a $55-billion-a-year industry and easily the most profitable business in America. Drug prices are a big part of the health care problem; drug companies are suddenly about as popular as the flu.

Now, with the government and the public demanding change, those companies are trying to defend themselves.

"Ask Mike what he would do if someone tried to take away his ulcer medicine," says a recent magazine ad sponsored by the American Pharmaceutical Coalition for Stupid Advertising. The ad shows a picture of Mike with his fists raised, implying that he would have to slap someone around, or perhaps take up puppetry—it's hard to tell which.

The irony is that nobody, not even Hillary Rodham Clinton, wants to take away Mike's medicine, although Mike may soon learn that he can't afford it anyway. Drug prices have gone up more than 150 percent during the last 10 years, and are still rising at three times the rate of inflation. No other legal business makes this kind of money.

Another full-page ad ran in 40 major newspapers, trying to justify these incredible price increases by saying that the money was used for important pharmaceutical research, and not just for marketing. Of course, it cost them half a million nonexperimental dollars to say so, but this is just pocket change compared with the more than $10 billion that they spend every year on promotion.

Drug manufacturers spend more for advertising than do beer companies, but have you ever seen a drug ad? A few years ago, unless you read doctor magazines or watched "Lifetime" on cable TV, the answer would have been no. Almost all of that money was spent, I am ashamed to say, on doctors.

Doctors are bombarded with drug advertising and merchandise from the start of medical school, when they receive their first free stethoscopes compliments of a major drug company. No one knows how many pens, sticky notes, plastic trinkets and free lunches doctors have received, each one an advertisement for some brand-name medicine. For a long time it was common to see respected physicians in highly specialized fields sporting 50-cent plastic pocket protectors with drug names on the front. Doctors were like top tennis players, performing as walking billboards for the products they used.

This behavior was so suspect that even members of Congress could see it was wrong. A few years ago they passed strict new laws controlling gifts to doctors. Now, to make up for it, the drug companies have started advertising directly to patients. This began with vague ads for hair restorers and female hormones, but now they even have commercials for prescription blood-pressure medicines during popular TV sitcoms.

The message "drugs are good" is being pounded into us all the time by these ads. They show us actors pretending to be sick people, who then pretend to be cured by the miracle of modern pharmaceuticals. "America has the best medicines in the world," they tell us, "thanks to the free-enterprise system. Wouldn't it be a shame if someone were to ruin it?" Some of the ads take an even more threatening tone: "Be nice to us, or we might just quit making drugs altogether, and then you'll be sorry."

The truth is that everyone knows prescription drugs are good—too good, in fact, for people to have to go without them. There are patients, generally older people, who are being forced to stretch out their pills—cutting them in half or doing without them altogether. I know this sounds Reaganesque, like anecdotes about Cadillac welfare queens, but there are people who must choose between buying

179

medicine and buying food. Even in my practice, in an average suburb, I've seen it happen.

It's going to take more than a few dumb ads to get drug companies off the hook. Real reform will mean giving up some of their tremendous profits to make sure everyone can afford the medicines they need. If not, you can expect to see some sort of mandatory price controls on drugs, whether or not the Clinton plan survives.

Maybe they could just take all the money they spend on doctors and advertising and use it to lower the price of their drugs. That way Mike could still have his ulcer medicine, and maybe have enough left over to buy himself a new puppet besides.

Otherwise, we will have the best medicines in the world sitting on shelves in our pharmacies, where they do no good at all.

Sick of the Lottery? Play Med Lotto

I noticed that the jackpot for the State Lottery was getting pretty large. I can always tell by the number of people waiting to buy tickets at the gas station. If the checkout line stretches back to the magazine rack, then I know the prize is over $10 million. If it reaches the Slurpee machine, it is approaching $20 million. If people are lined up all the way back to the video rentals, then the total is over $30 million and I have to make it home on the gas left in my tank.

Lottery fever is out of control. So is the cost of health care. Luckily, I've figured out a way to solve both problems.

It is amazing how fast the lottery has caught on. People were just waiting for an excuse to send their money to retired secretaries in Wisconsin. There are hardly any retired secretaries left in that state who have not become millionaires, thanks to Lotto. They may have to fly in some retired volunteers from other states just to keep it fair.

The odd thing is that gambling used to be a sin. I still think of it that way. The idea of organized gambling always makes me think of Marlon Brando in *The Godfather*. Because of this, I've never bought a lottery ticket, even though it means checking my bed each morning for severed horse heads.

Still, I seem to be the only one holding on to his change. Gambling is now a big moneymaker, even bigger than parking tickets during snow emergencies in Minnesota. We are now a nation of gambling junkies who will tear, peel, match, or rub any small piece of cardboard as long as it features a few dollar signs. They know someone has to win, and so they keep buying lottery tickets, even though their chances of winning are exactly the same as their chances of being the victim of a shark attack. Inland. While driving to work.

At the same time, the administration in Washington is trying to face the enormous crisis in health care. Whatever the result, it is clear that everyone is going to be asked to pitch in, paying more of the costs through taxes, higher insurance premiums, copayments, and the like.

Copayments already exist for some insurance plans, and needless to say, the concept has not been popular. People are used to their insurance paying their bills, and they have never been asked to turn over actual cash money at the doctor's office. Many people complain, and some refuse to pay the $5 or $10, leaving before they even see the doctor.

Why will people lay out so much money for a chance in the lottery, but not for a chance to stay healthy? I don't know, but I have figured out a solution. The answer? MedLotto.

Here's how it would work: People would flock to gas stations and liquor stores to buy tickets for MedLotto. The winning numbers will be read on TV, and the lucky ticket holders will receive a visit to the doctor of their choice. Different games will feature different medical specialties, allowing people to play for a chance at allergy shots or a gallbladder operation. Coupons for expensive tests or treatments will pile up until someone wins, and the really big jackpots will include complete physical exams, with X-rays, blood tests, and all.

People will still have a chance to select "Daily Three" numbers, but instead of random combinations they will be trying to guess the results of their cholesterol or blood sugar tests.

And once a month, in a gigantic jackpot lottery, some lucky winner will receive a "Get Out of the Hospital Free" card.

I think MedLotto makes a lot of sense. The government will soon be in the health care business anyway. We are going to see a lot of plans that are even goofier than this one, especially once Congress gets involved. MedLotto would be a way to provide good medical care and good, clean fun at the same time.

I know there will be a lot of people who say that MedLotto would never work. They will tell us that Americans will always have the right to see their own doctors whenever they want, despite their insurance company or the government. To these people, I have only one thing to say: Wanna bet?

Depo Provera—
Top Ten Excuses

Top 10 Reasons why the price of Depo-Provera, a female hormone injection made by Upjohn Co., suddenly jumped from $20 to $60 when it was approved for use as a new, long-acting form of birth control:

10. Upjohn's list of New Year's resolutions includes "Soulless Price Gouging."

9. Pay for celebrity endorsement from Madonna.

8. Need to fund extensive research, including several long-distance phone calls to some of the 90 other countries that have been using Depo-Provera as birth control for years.

7. C'mon, it's not like it costs men anything.

6. Overtime pay for laboratory geeks who stayed up late Tuesday night running important last-minute research tests.

5. Weed out people who merely enjoy receiving painful injections every three months.

4. Pay for important cost-analysis marketing surveys, including contacting several drugstores to see how much it costs for the same amount of birth control pills (hint: $60).

3. Pay for celebrity endorsement from Michael Jackson.

2. Promote bid to become the official injectable hormone of the 1996 Olympics.

And the No. 1 reason why the price of Depo-Provera suddenly jumped from $20 to $60:

1. Bill Clinton may be president, but with health reform dead, there's not a thing he can do about it.

Changing Insurance? Change Your Mind

Medical reports show that every January 40 percent of the people in the country are suffering from the flu, only they can't get to a doctor because the other 60 percent have recently changed health insurance.

It's like this every year. Doctors' offices are jammed with new patients who have just been forced to switch health plans, leaving them anxious and confused about who exactly is their doctor. In fact, between influenza and questions about new coverage, clinics are so busy that it may be easier to put a family member through medical school than to get through on the phone.

Not many people notice when their employers change insurance plans. The only obvious difference may be the color of that little benefits booklet they pass out in December. Who can tell when their medical coverage switches from "Medical One Gold Health Select" to "Medical Plus Choice Preferred Health One"?

Unfortunately, somewhere in that booklet, buried deep in the insurance gobbledygook, is the sentence that says the employees will have to change doctors—and people never realize it until it is too late.

A lot of people believe their last doctor was the best doctor in the world. It was their old doctor who cared for them as a child, set their broken bones, nursed them back from scarlet fever, gave them stitches when they bonked their head on the coffee table and took the time to listen to their dolls, like doctors do in Norman Rockwell paintings.

Now the insurance company wants them to pick a new doctor from an approved list. Although some would be obvious bad choices (such as the actual doctors named "Dr. Probe" and "Dr. Croak"), a list makes it hard to tell a kind, caring, Marcus Welby-type from a Jack Kevorkian.

The insurance changes can affect anybody, no matter how sick they are. Some patients are forced to switch cancer doctors in the middle of chemotherapy. Some people with heart problems have to quickly find new doctors, who will then tell them to avoid stress. If someone were undergoing emergency surgery on New Year's Eve, the insurance company would make the doctors stop in midoperation, cover the opening with a sheet and transport the patient to an approved hospital so new doctors could finish the job.

Luckily, most people are healthy. They wouldn't rush to the new doctor unless they needed refills on their medicines. Some people believe their previous insurance company might be generous and extend the prescription for a few months, giving them plenty of time to get to the doctor. Most companies have an 800 number for such problems as this. It takes a while to get through—the insurance people are busy too, between signing up new members and printing ads portraying Hillary Rodham Clinton as the devil—but they eventually reach someone who has the answer. That answer is usually, "Ha, ha," leaving the client no choice but to call the new clinic for an appointment.

Your last doctor would walk in, chat for a while, and write a new prescription. You didn't have to get embarrassed; you rarely even had to get undressed.

It won't be that easy now. This new doctor knows nothing about you. What if he or she doesn't believe you? Sure, you have the empty medicine bottle, but that's no real proof. Copies of medical records take months to arrive, and everyone looks nervous in a gown that is open in the back. You'll probably have to fake some sort of attack just to prove you really need the medicine.

It's enough to make you want to call your old doctor again, even if it means paying the bill yourself. Of course, the old clinic is jammed too, full of people telling the same stories about their old doctors. Some of them used to go to your new clinic, which means that every old doctor is now somebody else's new one. This arrangement makes sure nobody is happy.

When President Clinton announced his doomed Health Reform plan he was careful to reassure people that they would be able to pick their own doctors, even if they can't now. Maybe next time he could also get them to start the coverage later in the year, say maybe in June, when doctors are only treating softball injuries and an occasional sunburn.

Until then, you flu victims are on your own. Drink plenty of fluids, rest in bed and keep that 800 number handy, just in case.

Smoke Lies

A lot of people were shocked to learn how tobacco companies have been lying to us for years. They can't imagine how major corporations could stoop so low, evidently believing that they would draw the line at drug dealing, child endangerment, and mass murder.

Last year executives from seven major tobacco companies appeared before a congressional panel, where they stated for the millionth time that smoking is not bad for you. They had no idea what all the fuss was about. One of them even went on record as saying that cigarettes are "no worse than Twinkies or video games." Personally, I can't vouch for this, never having smoked a Twinkie.

A week later a bunch of top-secret documents were smuggled out of tobacco company vaults. They discussed research done 30 years ago by tobacco company scientists that clearly proved smoking causes cancer, heart attacks, and emphysema. It is now obvious that, no matter what they say, tobacco companies knew all along that their products are incredibly dangerous.

People and government officials were outraged at these revelations. Now the Food and Drug Administration (FDA) is threatening to regulate cigarettes like any hazardous drug; Congress is considering tough new regulations prohibiting smoking anywhere except inside abandoned nuclear containment generators. Retired politicians are saying that they would have banned smoking a long time ago if only they had known what tobacco companies were hiding.

While I'm happy that tobacco executives have finally been exposed as subhuman, lying scum, I don't understand all of this outrage. Really, anyone who is surprised by this latest round of deception just hasn't been paying attention.

Judging by the record, tobacco executives may be physically incapable of telling the truth. I bet that even during congressional hearings they were giving false names and switching the place cards around, just to keep people guessing. For years they have ignored a mountain of evidence against them, while reassuring their customers that smoking was glamorous and safe.

Take "light" cigarettes, for example. These were introduced years ago to make smokers feel better about the horrible risks they take every day. Light cigarettes are supposed to give you less of the tar and nicotine that tobacco companies refuse to say is harmful. Although the ads never come right out and say so, they all send the same message: "Light Cigarettes—taste great, less killing."

This is—you guessed it—a big, fat lie. "Light" cigarettes are no safer than any other brand; smoking light cigarettes to stay healthy is like using only low-caliber ammunition to shoot yourself. Blood levels of nicotine are sky-high in all smokers, regardless of the brand. The only time "light" nicotine levels are lower is on the special smoking machines they use for testing. (Many of these machines are now filing product liability suits.) Human smokers possess certain characteristics, like lips, that increase the amount of nicotine being delivered. Just by sucking harder they can turn lights into heavies, getting even more nicotine than regular brands.

Lies like this should be enough to send smokers storming into tobacco company offices, hunting down tobacco executives with torches like angry villagers in an old Frankenstein movie. With this in mind, is anyone really surprised by their ridiculous answers about smoking and health? Why would anyone ask them in the first place?

Thanks to these secret documents, tobacco people are having a hard time ignoring medical evidence produced by their own scientists. Instead, they have decided to ignore a different bunch of scientific evidence, this time dealing with addiction. While smoking may be somewhat unhealthy, they now say, it is really a matter of free choice. According to them, nicotine is not addictive. Anyone can quit, but no one should deprive them of their God-given right to choose to smoke.

Luckily, the FDA covered this when nicotine patches were introduced. Nicotine, as it turns out, is about as addictive as heroin or cocaine, although more people are able to stop using heroin than tobacco. That's why the patches require a prescription, forcing you to go to a doctor who can then try to talk you out of them.

About the only option left for the tobacco companies is to make a cigarette that doesn't contain nicotine. This has been possible for years, through a complicated process that eliminates the step where the manufacturers add it later. Of course, without the addictive properties of nicotine, no one would buy them. Not many people would spend the money just to smell bad and ruin their teeth.

Otherwise, cigarettes may soon become a prescription item, hidden behind the pharmacy counter instead of suspended above it in attractive displays featuring women in swimsuits hugging a camel. This would be one way to punish tobacco executives.

A better way would be to wait for their next ridiculous public appearance and then pelt them with Twinkies and video games, burying them in cream filling and "Sonic the Hedgehog" cartridges until they say they are sorry.

Even then, given their history, I wouldn't believe them.

Health Plans

It's not too late!

This is the basic underlying message of this book, which replaces the previous underlying message, "wait a half-hour after swimming."

While newspaper columns sometimes allowed to make you feel terrible, a book has to be uplifting. This last section is filled with important information on disease prevention, which gives you, the reader, a chance to stay healthy and allows you to write off the cost of the book as a medical expense.

Good Luck!

New New Years Resolutions

Every year millions of people across the country make New Year's resolutions. What this really means is one resolution—"lose weight"—split several million ways. If you listen carefully on New Year's Day you can hear the sound of Slim-Fast cans opening.

While this is a worthwhile goal, a lot of these people are bound to be disappointed. Expectations for this kind of thing are much too high. If some people aren't looking like Cher by February, they get depressed.

It makes more sense to set reasonable goals. Smaller resolutions are easier to stick with. There is enough to be depressed about in February.

Medical science can help. Here are some better New Year's resolutions, all based on sound medical principles that have nothing to do with weight. Clip this list and carry it with you today, telling everyone in a loud voice, "I resolve to:

"Eat more food"

The one sure way to lose weight—"eat less food"—is too hard for most people to stick with for very long. In fact, most people never make it past the half-time snacks during the Rose Bowl.

Instead, resolve to eat more food, but really horrible food. This takes away your appetite and makes you look forward to your next meal like you would to periodontal surgery.

The only problem is finding food that tastes worse than Slim-Fast. Most diet food today is a lot better than it used to be, and not everyone lives next to a Denny's.

To really make this work you would need to find some diet food from the '60s and '70s, like Melba toast or Metrocal, a nutritional diet supplement that could easily have been made from industrial waste.

"Move to Ecuador"

Science has shown that the Earth is not truly round, but bulges in the middle like many of its inhabitants. Things on the equator are farther from the center, and so they weigh less.

This proves that high school physics class was pretty darn important after all, and maybe you could have listened once in a while instead of writing notes and giggling in the back row, that is when you did show up instead of cutting class to sneak out and buy Ding Dongs at the 7-Eleven, only to find yourself hanging out with those rough kids from across town and eventually getting into a whole lot of trouble, and you know what I mean. But I digress.

"Grow"

Instead of losing weight, try gaining height. This is not as hard as it sounds, thanks to the emergence of bungee jumping as a popular pastime. Actual results may vary, depending on where you attach the cord.

"Wear vertical stripes"

This is based on the scientific principle that stripes make you look thinner, which doesn't work. What it does is let everyone know you are worried about your weight, prompting them to tell you things like, "What, did you lose some weight or something? You look great! Really!"

"Exercise"

Everyone knows they need more exercise, but they think this means taking up jogging. The odds that most people will become marathon runners are actually within a few decimal points of the odds that they will be nominated for pope.

Fortunately, medical science has shown that any exercise is useful for losing weight. Make it a part of daily life, even combining it with your other bad habits. Wherever you go, walk fast, even if just to the refrigerator. When you go to McDonald's, carry along enough coins to pay in pennies. Chew everything several extra times. Use really heavy silverware. And don't overlook important exercise opportunities such as skipping to work. You will be able to avoid many high-calorie meals as people stop inviting you over for dinner.

"Watch late-night television commercials for fat-burning grapefruit gut-buster diets"

Hysterical laughter burns calories.

"Wear a hat"

It is a well-known scientific fact that you lose between 10 percent and 90 percent of your body heat from your head, depending on whose mother is being quoted. While it won't make you any thinner, at least this resolution should be easier to stick to. Remember, it gets pretty cold in February.

Lifetime Warranty Runs Out at 40

A lot of people worry about getting older, just because their bodies fall apart and they are that much closer to death.

This is silly. There is no reason to worry about what is going to happen when you are 60 or 70, not with so much to worry about at 40.

I am not there yet, but I have already seen the road signs of deterioration warning me to ease over into the slow lane of middle age on the four-lane tollway of life.

I chew my food more carefully now. It takes days to recover from such physically demanding tasks as cleaning the gutters. I pay attention to commercials about gum disease. I don't jog with younger people because I'm afraid they will be bothered by the noises coming from my knees. It's becoming clear that my body will someday be recalled by the manufacturer.

I know I'm not the only one who feels this way. People come into my office every day complaining about this. Anyone alive during any part of the Eisenhower administration is starting to feel this same gradual decline; the baby boomers are getting older.

"I can't hear like I used to," they say, or "My back gave out while lifting . . . a pencil."

We are all slower, heavier and generally much more like our parents than we would like.

"You don't understand," they plead, "I used to be able to stay up all night building beer-can pyramids and still be sharp for midterms in the morning, and after only 13 cups of coffee."

It's my job to let them know that, sadly, those days are over. The bloom is off the boom. "Nothing's wrong," I tell them. "You are just getting older." No one is ever happy to hear this, particularly when I add the part about eating more fiber.

To understand the aging process you first have to realize what happens to other organic material on the planet. Remember the time you unknowingly dropped a wiener and it rolled under the refrigerator? Remember how it looked when you finally found it, several weeks after having the house fumigated?

This same process is going on in our bodies all the time. We are all in a constant state of "going bad," some parts faster than others.

Luckily, our bodies are continually making new cells to replace the ones that fall off and end up under the fridge. We manage to keep up with the decay for years, even through the incredible demands of puberty, but sooner or later things start to slide.

At 40 we are suddenly able to replace only the most important cells, like heart and small intestine cells, while things like knees and eyes have to fend for themselves. Fat cells do particularly well after 40, and our bodies will often try to use them as replacements for other parts, passing them off as a new chin or set of thigh muscles.

There are other changes too. Doctors never go by calendar age during physical exams, relying instead on other, more precise physiological indicators of middle age.

Like eyebrow hair. Most men have perfectly normal brows, until one day when they suddenly sprout several long, stiff hairs that make them look like giant lobsters from space. Trimming only makes them thicker. Soon they are extending back over the forehead, trying to catch the quickly receding hairline.

Ear hair also appears during this period, causing many men to wonder when hair will show up on their eyeballs and other smooth organs. These hairs are long enough for everyone to notice, but too short to use for the popular "comb-over" method of covering bald spots, which, according to my friend's uncle Rob, turns the scalp into a large bar code. People will do anything to combat this growth, even to the point of using dangerous rotary "personal grooming" devices that, in careless hands, can easily carve an entirely new ear canal.

Still, it's hard to blame them. Middle age is difficult to accept. Most of us are not even ready to be grown-ups yet, much less old people. Some of us are just pretending to be adults because we have important jobs.

198

Luckily, not everyone has to suffer through this phase of life. Every so often you meet people in their 80s who still run marathons while managing their own corporations, between doing volunteer work at children's hospitals and flying to Rome to perform their latest violin concerto before the pope.

These people are an inspiration, and they always bring one thought to mind: Maybe next year I can get one of them to come and clean my gutters.

Where There's Smoking, There's Fire

I love it when new antismoking articles come out, like the recent study that showed smoking causes cataracts. It turns out that when they told us, "If you don't stop, you'll go blind," they were talking about smoking.

I often clip out headlines like this, carrying them around for a few days to show patients and people at work. "Well, that ought to do it," I tell them happily. "Surely no one could possibly keep smoking now."

They just look at me and shake their heads. I know what they're thinking. They think I don't understand smoking, and of course they're right. To me, smoking makes about as much sense as, well, putting something in your mouth and then lighting it on fire.

This happened again when I first heard about the new "sin tax" on cigarettes. President Clinton asked for a tax of $2 a pack to help pay for the cost of health care reform. This seemed reasonable to me, especially since smokers are the ones who will be using up lots of our health care.

Other people don't see it that way. Many of them were upset, especially tobacco farmers, tobacco lobbyists, and tobacco-puppet senators like Jesse Helms. These people are worried that the tax will cut down on "free trade." Personally, I'm worried that $2 a pack is not nearly enough.

I've always been amazed by the things people can tolerate to keep smoking. Smoking makes you smell bad, stains your teeth yellow, and turns your skin into beef jerky. It eats away at your lungs inside your chest, and eventually causes your heart to seize up like a rusty fuel pump on a '68 Buick.

Unfortunately, except for the smell, these effects take a while to appear. Nobody realizes how dangerous smoking is until it is too late. It would almost be better if some of the more serious effects occurred immediately—say, that someone puts a lit cigarette in their mouth and boom, their head explodes. Let them try to explain that in the box on the side of the package.

Of course, whatever they printed in the box, the tobacco companies would still deny it. They deny everything, even the warning labels on their own products. Even now, they maintain that smoking does not cause health problems, according to their own highly trained research scientists.

There is just no "hard evidence," their lobbyists tell legislators. "We'll let you know. In the meantime, here, have some more money."

So far, civil courts have not been able to blame cigarette manufacturers for the harm they do, but it's just a matter of time. On that day you can expect tobacco companies to release important new research showing that cancer really isn't so bad after all, and besides, there's really no evidence that dying ever hurt anyone.

These same companies are constantly trying to recruit new smokers, largely because the old ones keep dying off. That's why their billboard advertisements feature cartoon characters bearing a suspicious resemblance to Barney the dinosaur. They know if they can get kids to take a few puffs they will be hooked, thanks to the incredibly addictive nature of tobacco, which is roughly the same as a heroin-laced chocolate Ding Dong soaked in brandy.

With this in mind, it is hard to believe that $2 is really going to make much difference. Even so, the tax has been violently opposed by groups like the Tobacco Institute, a place where people enroll to study economic trends while smoking. These people say they are worried that a smoking tax would be unfair to poor people, who should have the same right to hazardous, toxic products as anyone else.

This kind of whining quickly started chipping away at the new tax. When last seen, it was already down to about 90 cents a pack, and dropping fast. The final version may only ask smokers to make a voluntary contribution to their local health department, while calling for mandatory recycling of the plastic wrapping.

There is only one answer: Just say no. We need to turn our federal anti-drug forces on North and South Carolina, just as we did with Colombia. The Army could set up an embargo on the interstate, preventing tobacco trucks from leaving. The Air Force could begin defoliant spraying of all tobacco fields. The FBI could run elaborate sting operations to capture idiotic, bloated legislators like Helms, imprisoning them in luxury penthouse apartments with state-of-the-art entertainment systems, from which they could escape at will.

Better yet, we could line them all up and stick dry leaves in their mouths. To help them pass the time, they could take turns setting each other on fire.

Chewing the Fat about Cholesterol

People are tired of hearing about cholesterol, and I don't blame them. Most of us have no idea what we eat during an average day, and the last thing we need is another expert explaining what is bad for us.

Besides that, they keep changing the rules. Remember oat bran? Didn't you eat enough oat bran muffins to fill a silo? Well, too bad, because now they've decided that oat bran is no better than any other bran, which means it is about the same as not eating at all only you have to go to the bathroom more often.

I don't blame people for having trouble with the cholesterol thing, but I think they owe it to themselves to try again. Anyone can learn a few simple facts that can give them a better grip on the problem. Here is a clear, easy-to-follow explanation of cholesterol in basic English:

The word cholesterol is taken from the Latin chole, which means "bile," and esterol, meaning "substance that will clog all your arteries and cause your heart to wear out before your radial tires do." The basic thing to understand about cholesterol is this: Any at all is bad, and more is worse.

The cholesterol you eat, although it is bad, is only part of the story. Your body is making new cholesterol all the time. When you decide to eat less of it, your body decides to make more. Basically, this is like knitting a rope so that you can use it to hang yourself. This should prove, in case anyone skipped puberty, that the workings of the human body are indeed mysterious.

To make things even more complicated, this total cholesterol is then broken up into different components. These are called lipoproteins, from the words lipo, which means "fat," and protein, or "for the teenager." This is, of course, the time in life when most people move away from their parents and learn to survive on nothing more than microwave pizzas and Hostess Twinkies.

LDL, or Long Distance Lipoprotein, is the really scary kind of cholesterol. These fat molecules set up tiny tollbooths in the arteries, collecting a surcharge on blood traveling toward the heart. After many years they become even more demanding, asking you to "deposit 2 Oreos for another three minutes of heartbeat." Like any long-distance company, they can cut you off suddenly at any time, only it's not just the line that goes dead.

If your doctor is on the cutting edge of medicine, he may decide to order an apo-protein test. This name, which means "above the average protein," refers to the cost of the test, which is somewhere between dinner for two at Sardi's and purchasing an oceangoing Hovercraft. Most people have a hard time understanding what apo-proteins are, but don't worry about them, because doctors don't know either.

Is it necessary to understand the biochemical pathways that our bodies use to break down these dangerous fat molecules? No. At least, I sure hope not, because I forgot all that stuff years ago.

No, what is important is to use these principles to decide which foods are safe to eat, as in the following examples:

Baked potato with butter—bad
Double cheeseburger with extra mayo—terrible
16-ounce rib-eye steak with mushrooms and gravy—horrible
2 1/2 ounces of lean turkey breast on piece of lettuce—bad

See how easy it is? Now you are ready to put this knowledge into practice, following a careful eating plan that will keep your cholesterol under control while allowing you to enjoy a variety of interesting foods, as long as they all contain some sort of bark:

Breakfast—four small twigs from the ground near the back corner of the house
Lunch—Some grass clippings, with a sprinkling of mulch and a lemon wedge

Dinner—Hay (a free food) and plenty of it, with a small
spinach salad and a piece of fruit
Snack—More twigs, or perhaps a small glass of mineral water
Snack after everyone else goes to bed—Slim-Jim

With this kind of basic knowledge and careful planning, everyone can learn to keep their cholesterol under control. And who knows? You may even live longer. Either way, it will certainly seem longer.

Diet Plans That Shrink the Wallet

People everywhere want to lose weight, so I thought it would be a good idea to take a look at some popular weight-loss plans.

Remember, body weight is affected by two things: 1) the amount of body there is to weigh, and 2) the downward gravitational pull of the Earth. Experts are divided on which one is easier to change. Because I have forgotten most of my high-school physics, we'll have to focus on those plans that promise to decrease body size.

The Famous Losers Plans

These are the diet plans named after famous people whom you never heard of, who used to weigh a lot but don't anymore. You can see their advertisements in magazines and newspapers, often next to the horoscopes. They always feature a "before" photo of a customer, taken with a disposable camera in dim light from a distance of a half-mile, showing the vague outline of someone wearing sweat pants. There is also an "after" photo, a professional glamour shot of a smiling, slender person in Spandex. They are holding the old sweat pants, which now look like they could accommodate the Popeye balloon from the Macy's parade. The famous losers all say that they tried the other plans, wasting thousands of dollars before developing their own weight-loss systems. Now they offer their methods to others, in an effort to get some of the money back.

The Nutra-Opti-Slim-Reducing-Protein-Fast Diet Plans

These plans are for people who want to lose weight in the privacy of their own homes. The idea is to purchase many cases of pow-

206

dered brown sludge at the grocery store, and to eat the sludge instead of actual food. You lose weight because nobody can eat very much of the stuff and still have any appetite at all. You could do the same thing without the sludge, just skipping a meal or two each day, but it would be slightly less nutritional.

Health Clubs of the Stars

What do Shari Belafonte, Sheena Easton, and Raquel Welch have in common? That's right: They have no jobs. At least, not until recently. Now they are on TV with several other celebrities, promoting a variety of health and exercise clubs. If you want to look like Cher, they say on TV, all you have to do is work out for 30 minutes every other day. This is a little misleading, in that it doesn't even mention the $450,000 worth of plastic surgery, besides tattoos. Still, it is not much to ask of someone who wants to lose weight, as long as they have no job.

The Black Hole Diet Plan

A lot of people stick with this plan for years, even though it never works. "I never eat a thing," they tell their friends, "But I keep gaining weight." Their friends nod knowingly, remembering the time last week when they saw them down half a cheesecake and a Snickers bar before lunch.

These people believe they are exempt from the Law of Conservation of Matter, which states that Snickers bars are not allowed to disappear into thin air. It is important to remember that black holes are the most massive things in the universe, and that no one wants to end up in second place.

Late-Night TV Plans

Here are the really interesting weight-loss schemes. On late-night television you can see people who eat 17 grapefruits a day; machines that strap onto your stomach and let you exercise while you sleep; old movie stars squeezing large metal springs with their thighs. Do any of these things make sense to you? If so, you will probably not be losing any pounds in the near future, unless you happen to live in England.

The Common Sense Plan

Eat less food. That's it, the whole plan. Eat a little less if you want to lose a little, a lot less if you can't even remember exactly where your feet are located. This can mean using a smaller plate, or switching from a trough to a plate if necessary. Trade in the fork for chopsticks, pull an uncomfortable Swedish chair up to the table, cook food you don't like, watch CNN coverage of Congress during dinner—however you manage to do it, it will work. It can even apply to specific food groups, like the "things in crinkly bags" group or the "Hostess cream-filled" group. Eat less food, lose more weight. When combined with an occasional walk around the block, it can't miss.

Which of these weight-loss plans is right for you? It depends on the individual, but generally, if you are a human organism on the planet Earth who sometimes drives a car or wears stockings, then the last plan is probably the one for you. Consult your doctor if there is any question, and be sure to bring along that new "Fat Buster" you ordered from the late-night TV commercial. That kind of thing can really break up a busy day in the office.

New Food Labels Tell Too Much

The FDA has released its new guidelines for food labels, and I know I speak for all of us when I say, please pass the low-cal fat-free decaffeinated low-sodium artificial mocha-flavored frozen yogurt.

People haven't always needed government labels on food. In caveman times, people ate whatever they could catch.

Unfortunately, modern supermarkets have made it much too easy to catch things like Twinkies and Polish sausages, so we need the government to tell us what is safe to eat. This is in keeping with its continuing mission of protecting us from things that are bad for us. After all, it would be silly to regulate things like lawn darts while letting chocolate eclairs run around free.

Although the old food labels seem confusing, they were actually quite easy to interpret, assuming you knew the official code. For example, take a look at these common phrases found on supermarket shelves today:

"**Low Fat**" Translation: Contains less fat than fat itself.

"**Reduced Fat**" Less fat than it used to have, at least as measured by molecular biologists using powerful electron microscopes.

"**Lo Fat**" Less fat as measured by cretins who can't spell.

"**Diet**" Flavor-challenged and/or taste-impaired.

"**Low Cal**" Contains very few calories when eaten in portions the size of purely theoretical particles.

"**Cholesterol Free**" Contains no cholesterol. May still contain enormous globs of fat, which your body will turn into cholesterol before you even finish swallowing.

The new labels take a much more scientific approach. They compare everything to a "sample daily diet" containing 2,000 calories and 65 grams of fat. According to government research, this is what Americans should eat in an average day, even though many of us

209

eat this many calories while waiting for the pizza delivery man to show up with our actual meal.

They also simplify the code, making companies follow at least some rules when using certain words. Anything labeled "light" must have at least 50 percent less fat than other, more massive versions. "More" will mean 10 percent, not just a few molecules more. Although they stop short of recommending mandatory prison terms for the use of words like "lite," "lo," or "kwik 'n' e-z microwav snaks," they are still a major breakthrough for nutritional ethics.

Plus, they focus on fat content, which is something that people can understand. The old labels were full of confusing things like percentages and chemical names like "2-hydroxy monosorbitrontium glutamate," used to produce the pleasing, rubbery texture of Hostess Sno Balls. Nobody has ever seen a riboflavin, so why should they care how many of them are in microwave corn dogs? Fat is something you could hold in your hands, although it would be gross. Everyone knows fat is bad. With the new labels, it's just a matter of adding up the numbers.

I think they should make the labels even simpler, using phrases like "Contains more fat than a congressional payroll," or "Eating this is like having reverse liposuction." Or maybe they could list the amount of exercise needed to burn it off, like this label for French Silk Chocolate Pie: "Begin jogging in place immediately after eating, holding two steam irons and drinking nothing but warm Fresca. Stop when blood sugar returns to normal or at the next lunar eclipse, whichever comes first."

Most people really only need to know one thing—whether something is good or bad for them.

Does anyone really need to know precisely how many grams of fat are in Sara Lee Original Strawberry Cream Cheesecake? With "cake" and "cheese" featured prominently in the title you can bet that the fat count will be right up there with onion rings and Haagen-Dazs.

Maybe there should be just three different food labels: 1) a green label that says "Healthy, Eat Anytime," 2) a yellow one for "Medium Healthy, Eat Once in a While," and 3) the red "WARNING!

Dangerous, To be eaten only when absolutely necessary, such as after blind dates or IRS tax audits."

Either that, or we could just go back to the system where we can eat whatever we catch, which is fine with me. With the proper spiral, you can teach a friend to throw Twinkies a good ten yards.